got cancer?

(spring break gone bad)

Order this book online at www.trafford.com
or email orders@trafford.com

Most Trafford titles are also available at major online book retailers.

Note for Librarians: A cataloguing record for this book is available from Library
and Archives Canada at www.collectionscanada.ca/amicus/index-e.html

Printed in Victoria, BC, Canada.

ISBN: 978-1-4251-6448-5 (sc)
ISBN: 978-1-4269-1433-1 (dj)
ISBN: 978-1-4251-6449-2 (e-book)

*Our mission is to efficiently provide the world's finest, most comprehensive
book publishing service, enabling every author to experience success.
To find out how to publish your book, your way, and have it available
worldwide, visit us online at www.trafford.com*

Trafford rev. 8/3/2009

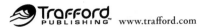 www.trafford.com

North America & international
toll-free: 1 888 232 4444 (USA & Canada)
phone: 250 383 6864 ✦ fax: 812 355 4082

James J. Gaudio

got cancer?

(spring break gone bad)

This book is dedicated to my wife, Eva, and to the medical personnel whose efforts saved my life.

Contents

Introduction

I AM A HIGH school science teacher, chemistry, principally. At times, I like to take a break from the rigors of academic learning by telling my chemistry students a story. Story telling is a quick and easy way to give the students (and me) a bit of a rest as we travel through what, at times, can seem like an endless school year.

As it happens, I am bald. Of course, my students never let me forget this fact. Again, it is a long school year, and I am a very demanding teacher. So, by letting the kids have license to tease me about something, I give them a means by which to gain a measure of revenge against me. I say this because, as their teacher, I hold the power to dictate what is to be done, how it is to be done and so forth. Having the power to tease me about something allows them to avoid feeling completely powerless in our relationship. Besides, I like a certain amount of banter in my classroom, so long as it remains civil.

One of my best stories concerns how I had to come to terms with the inevitability of going bald. By my early twenties, I knew for certain that my hairline was receding. I was sure that I would be lucky to make it into my early thirties with any significant amount of hair on my head. In fact, had I been able to strike a deal with the devil that would have guaranteed delaying my going bald until after my twenties,

I would have eagerly accepted. I had become obsessed with going bald. It seemed I was too often staring into some mirror speculating about "how much time I had left." I also found myself surreptitiously comparing my hairline with that of some man I socially encountered, and feeling envious if his fate was likely hairier than mine. I had become pathetically obsessed with my going bald. It was as if I had fallen into a vanity-induced coma. How could I escape the grip of this obsession, an obsession rooted in worry over the fate of my pate?

Clearly, a concern with personal appearance is a part of life, and teenagers are certainly very sensitive to matters pertaining to one's looks. Consequently, my chemistry students are typically very eager to hear how it was that I came to terms with such a drastic and socially undesirable change in my appearance. Baldness posed serious implications. For example, some student invariably offers that once a guy is bald, his dating life is shot, kaput, over. Of course, the kid is dead-on in his or her observation. This is to say that the main reason I was so worried about my hair was that I was concerned with being much less attractive to the opposite sex without it. Even though I was married during the peak (or perhaps the depth) of my obsession with hair, I was worried that my wife would lose interest in the bald version of me. Of course such thinking was an insult to my wife's love for me, but I was not thinking very clearly at the time.

How in the world would I ever move past this silly obsession?

Enter my father.

As it was, my father was bald, and had been since about his mid-twenties. He was very aware of my concern with baldness. I am certain that he was hoping that I would grow out of this "phase" and get on with my life. My father was a practical minded man. To be sure, Dominick Frank Gaudio, the seventh child of eight born to Italian immigrants, raised through the depression, a combat veteran of World War II, a hard bargaining union man, a veteran of gut-wrenching political campaigns, had no time for superficial nonsense. In fact, I had the suspicion that dad was getting fed up with my obsession with my hair. My suspicion was confirmed in spades one afternoon during a visit with him.

I happened to be in the vicinity of my folks' neighborhood one summer afternoon, and decided to drop in for a visit. My parents and I were not getting along very well at this time in my life. This is probably why my father and I ended up talking outside on his front lawn. He probably wanted me separated from my mother in order to reduce the chance for friction. I cannot remember what he and I were talking about, but during the course of conversation, I impulsively decided to ask something like, "Dad, did you ever think about doing something about being bald?"

He made no oral reply to my question, at least at first. Instead, he gave me a look that reeked of a father's disappointment in his son. Then, shaking his head slightly with his eyes closed, he slowly dropped his head until his chin was near his chest. Such was his exasperation that he was having difficulty even looking at me.

In that moment, I imagine he was thinking something like, "In all these years, haven't I taught this kid to understand the difference between what is important and what is unimportant in this life?" In the next moment, he jerked his head upward so as to be looking at me eyeball to eyeball, and then he really let me have it.

"Wake up, son! Get your head in the game! Don't you understand that had I been standing in the mirror counting the hairs on my head, none of us would have eaten? You play the hand you're dealt in this life, and bald-ain't-that-tough-a-hand!"

That was all he said. That was all he needed to say. He turned his back to me and stomped off.

I stood stunned. I neither moved nor spoke for a few seconds. When juxtaposed against my father's pragmatism, my silly enslavement to a concern as superficial as hair loss was embarrassing. I felt like a mental or emotional weakling. I was acting like a boy. The old man was right yet again. It was time I started to act like a man.

It is not my intent to give the impression that I was completely cured of my obsession by my father's blast. However, his explosion of very adverse criticism did spin me around. Like someone who had been hopelessly wandering in a dense fog, I locked on to his censure and used it to navigate myself clear.

When telling this story to my students, I emphasize at the end that its moral is the need to develop in life an ability to distinguish between matters of significance and those of insignificance. Acknowledging that hair loss for a woman is probably different, I point out that for a man, going bald is as painful as he chooses to make it, or as painful as he allows Madison Avenue to make it. I caution that going bald is one thing. It is altogether different than feeling ill, going to the doctor and having the "c-word" come up in the diagnosis. Baldness is a matter of vanity. Cancer is a matter of life and death. The two matters are clearly unequal.

Over my thirteen years of teaching, I told this story to many students. I never calculated that my life was fated to serve as the chalkboard on which the aforementioned inequality would be illustrated.

As it was, fate caught up with me during spring break of the '06 - '07 school year. The following pages contain, for the most part, a blow-by-blow, diary-like account of the events constituting my induction into the cancer patients' club.

CHAPTER ONE

Signals from the Stairs

MY CLASSROOM IS on the second (top) floor and at the south end of my school building. It is about as far away from the teachers' parking lot as a classroom can be. This trek is made even more demanding by my need to tote a very heavy computer case (used as my not-so-brief briefcase) to and from work on a daily basis. In fact, this case is about the size of a small suitcase. Like many suitcases, it is equipped with wheels and telescoping pull handle. I love it. Up until two years ago, I had used a lift-and-carry type case. Ugh! My wheeled case is much superior, as long as the surface that must be traversed is reasonably smooth. Of course, such a wheeled case offers no advantage when one has to deal with stairs.

Upon my entry into the school building, it was my habit to ascend the two flights of stairs on the north end of the building. These stairs lead to the building's second floor. The lower flight consists of sixteen steps from the first floor to the landing. The upper flight consists of fourteen steps connecting the landing to the second floor. With or without a load, these stairs can offer an opportunity to test one's physical condition. Accordingly, I would sometimes make the climb as fast as I could, just to take measure of my conditioning. Unfortunately, a day came when I would no longer have to try to make the climb difficult. On that day, and much to my chagrin, I discovered that even a slow paced, methodical climb up these stairs became an endeavor that pushed me to my physical limits. The stairs were telling me something, but I did not want to listen.

I am the type of person who works very earnestly at maintaining my physical condition. Truthfully, I exercise almost every day of the year, and very rigorously. To illustrate, on one day my exercise consists of hard riding a stationary exercise bike, mixed with punching and kicking a forty-pound heavy bag. Such a session typically runs for forty-five minutes. On the following day, I again use the stationary bike, but I do pushups and a form of weight lifting instead of working the bag. Again, the session runs for forty-five minutes. Even if I am out of town and away from the gym (i.e., my garage), I will walk for miles at a time on a daily basis, often mixing in pushups, periodically. Therefore, on that day in mid-February when my morning ascent of the school's stairs left me feeling like I was on the brink of death, I was stunned. By the time I cleared the stairs from the first floor to the landing, I knew that something was different. By the time I cleared the flight from the landing to the second floor, I knew something was wrong. My bag and legs felt as if they were made of lead, and my legs ached, too. I was very short of breath and light-headed. My heart raced, and I could feel its beat pounding in my head. I wondered if I might faint. I had to take a moment to recover. What was this about?

In terms of physical endurance, I did not even recognize myself. I could never have expected that ascending these stairs would leave me feeling so depleted. Finding myself feeling so defeated at the top of the stairs was as shocking as if I had looked into a mirror and seen the reflection of a complete stranger.

Once on the second floor, I did manage to recover from this stunning turn of events fairly quickly. With little ado, I extended the pull-handle on my case and began pulling my case southward along the upper floor, heading to my classroom. There were students along my route, but I could only absent-mindedly exchange morning greetings with those who offered them to me. My mind was far more concerned with an acceptable explanation for what I had just experienced. Was I catching some sort of bug? Was my struggle on the stairs just something weird, an anomaly? "There must be some simple explanation," I thought. I resolved to put the matter out of my mind.

The first two periods of my workday were chemistry classes, specifically, honors chemistry. Teaching this course is very consuming, so I had no problem keeping my resolve to avoid thinking about my earlier trouble with climbing the stairs. The third period of the day was my plan period. Soon after the start of this period, I would typically take advantage of an opportunity to use the restroom. For various reasons, I avoided the boys' student restrooms as if they were the plague itself. My preference was to use a men's restroom near the principal's office. This preference meant that I had to go downstairs to the first floor. Downstairs I went. Of course, going down meant I would have to go back up. My resolve was weakening.

After taking care of personal matters, checking my mailbox and exchanging pleasantries with various office personnel, I headed for the building's centrally located stairs with a considerable amount of trepidation. The same laws of physics that assaulted me earlier, awaited me once again. This time up, however, I would be without my bag. To simulate earlier conditions, I decided to take the steps two at a time and in a sprint. Up I went. Before I had reached the landing, I was feeling uncomfortable. By the time I made it to the top of the second flight, I found myself needing to scale back my effort. I now knew that the earlier episode was not an anomaly. There was definitely something wrong with me. I took consolation in the "I must have some kind of bug" theory.

Climbing stairs continued to beat me up on a daily basis for about the next three weeks. As my ability to climb stairs continually worsened, I came to dread them. I began to feel like a kid who had to face some bully on a daily basis. Even the two minor staircases in my home had become troublesome. I was beginning to lose confidence in the "I must have a bug" theory.

One evening in the middle of March, my wife, Eva, asked me to take a walk with her. Our intention was to cover a total distance of about eight city blocks, and to do so at a fairly brisk pace. "No big deal," I thought. Well, I was wrong. We were no more than two or three minutes into our paces, and I felt like I might have a heart attack. I said nothing to Eva because I did not want to alarm her, but *I* was plenty alarmed. Normally, I would have barely qualified an outing such as this as being a legitimate exercise session, yet I had to strain to keep up with *her!* This was very strange. A new theory was becoming necessary. About a week later, my need for a new theory was confirmed when I went on a similar walk with a visiting friend. In so doing, I felt as bad as I had when walking with Eva, if not worse. I could not quite believe my current response to simple activity like climbing stairs and brisk walking. In the past, I had hiked and bicycled well above tree line without feeling so sickly. "What was happening to me?" I kept wondering with mounting annoyance.

Another puzzlement about my trouble was that I continued to exercise in my gym with less difficulty than I experienced when ascending stairs or taking brisk walks. This was very strange to me, although I had to admit to myself that my exercise sessions had become less energetic. I also noticed that I was becoming increasingly reluctant to do my exercises after I arrived home from work. But my decrease in energy and my desire to be lazy could be easily explained: I was deep into the school year, and I was rapidly approaching my fifty-sixth birthday. An aging teacher well into the school year could be expected to be low on energy and feeling a little lazy. I still lacked, however, an explanation for why it was that my workouts were not killing me, but brisk walking and stair climbing were. Back to the drawing board I went.

Identifying my problem was rather simple, from my point of view: My trouble with brisk walking and stair climbing meant that I had lost my aerobic conditioning. My question was, "*How* did this loss happen?" I was surprised at the ease with which I was able to come up with a sensible explanation. I concluded that there were two principal factors leading to my aerobic decline. The first was the fact that my exercise bike had been in a state of disrepair for months. Over this span of time, I could not use it for peddling while standing up with the flywheel clamp set at high resistance. Using the exercise bike in this fashion was how I would mimic climbing a steep hill. Clearly, my exercise routine had lost much of its aerobic rigor due to an inadequate exercise bike. The second factor was related to our family dog, Boots. About seven months prior to my troubles, I had stopped walking her. Over the years, I would walk her on a daily basis for forty to fifty minutes per session. To make sure she got a good workout, I kept my pace at no lower than one hundred and thirty strides per minute. However, by the fall of '06, Boots was well over eleven years old, and her serious walking days were clearly behind her. I resorted to simply strolling her for ten to fifteen minutes per session. These strolls were so sissified relative to our old style of walking that I did not even consider them to be a legitimate form of exercise.

Terrific! I had it all figured out. I only needed to change my exercise routine such that a significant aerobic component would be reintroduced. My problems would soon be behind me.

With about ten days remaining in March, I changed my exercise regimen. Each day's session was to begin with thirty minutes of my normal gym exercises. Immediately following, I bolted the gym walking at one hundred and thirty paces, or more, per minute. My objective was to maintain such a pace for a full twenty minutes. I was able to achieve this objective in a little over a week's time, although by the end of such a walk I was really pooped. The good news was that the time I needed to recover after such walking was lessening with each session.

My confidence in my progress was such that I had even blended a little jogging in with the fast-pace walking. Honesty compelled me, nonetheless, to acknowledge that the walking and jogging still left me with a strange feeling in my chest and a pounding in my head. I also continued to notice that I seemed always to be tired, even to the point of wondering if I were, in fact, suffering from fatigue. I even wondered about pneumonia a time or two, but ruled it out since I displayed none of the typical symptoms. If everything else were not enough, I began to notice a new problem in the mornings: The calves of my legs would want to severely cramp when I stretched my legs upon first waking up.

In spite of all my efforts, I was unable to truly fix myself. Something was wrong within me, and a climb up any staircase would quickly reveal the presence, although not the nature, of my mysterious malady.

During my weeks of struggle, I said little about the details to Eva. The only thing that I would commonly mention to her was that I always seemed to feel tired. I even stated to her at one point that I was getting tired of always talking to her about how tired I felt. Eventually, Eva decided the time for complaint had passed and that I needed to see a doctor.

Over the years, Eva learned that suggesting that I see a doctor could be tricky. This was true even when I knew in my heart that I should see a doctor. My wife needed to wait until the time was right for offering this suggestion. She deemed that time to be Wednesday of spring break week. I had been feeling very tired and irritable that day. While eating supper, I also told Eva about the troubles I had been experiencing with walking and stairs. Shortly after supper, Eva asked if I would consider making a doctor's appointment to find out what was going on with me. In knee-jerk fashion, I said, "No."

Eva said nothing in reply. She had been down this road before and figured that I would likely come to my senses if left alone for a while. She was right. Later that evening, I agreed to let our family doctor look me over. In her willingness to make things as easy as she could for me, Eva promised to call the clinic soon after it opened on Thursday morning and make an appointment for me to see Dr. James Freudenburg. When she called, Eva was able to get me an appointment for ten-thirty of that very morning. I had assumed that I would have to wait until the next week for an appointment. I could not know it at the time, but it was very lucky for me that I got in to see the doctor so soon. As it turned out, my condition was perilous and worsening by the minute.

Over a period of about six weeks, I had come to see stairs as my nemesis. As it turns out, they had been signaling me warnings about my worsening health all along. I had just been too ignorant to properly interpret the signals.

At a little past ten on Thursday morning, April 5, 2007, I left for my appointment with Dr. Freudenburg. I had no idea what lay ahead. And I mean *no* idea.

CHAPTER TWO

What's Up (with Me), Doc?

B Y CONSENTING TO see a doctor, I had officially acknowledged that there was something wrong with me, something that I alone could not fix. Still, as I drove to Dr. Freudenburg's office, I was more concerned with the amount of my spring break vacation that I would have to burn on medical matters than I was with the nature of my medical problem. I would soon learn that, for me, spring break was over, at least in any recreational sense.

A clinic within a couple miles drive of my home is the location of Dr. Freudenburg's office. This clinic is always quite busy, but I have found it to be efficient in its operations. True to form, I whizzed through the check-in station. Next up, a brief stop at the blood pressure and pulse station. After that, I was headed to the waiting area. Once there, I barely had time to grab a magazine worth looking over and to select a seat away from the flow of traffic when I heard "James Gaudio" being called from behind me. One of the doctor's staff was calling for me. I cannot recall that I recognized this woman, but she was nice and, after taking my weight, soon had me seated in one of the examination rooms. I removed my hooded sweatshirt and cap upon entry. I then took a seat in one of the two chairs available while placing the clothing I had removed in the other. As I was taking a loose inventory of the various items in the room, a nurse came in with a folder, my folder. She asked what brought me in that day. It probably took me a minute to ninety seconds to give a synopsis of my symptoms. She made notations without making comment as I spoke. Within two minutes, she was on her way out, assuring me that the doc would be in shortly. I continued with my inventory of the room's stuff.

I could hear that there was considerable bustle in the hall outside my room's closed door. The place seemed pretty busy that morning. This would seem to reinforce my feeling that I got an appointment on the same day my wife called for one due to a cancellation. I heard the doc's voice. I did not pay as much attention to what he was saying as I was in trying to determine if he was stopping outside my room on his way in. He was not. I would have to wait a little longer before seeing him. I started to study a large photograph hanging on the west wall. The subject of the photo was some person caught in a moment of obvious enjoyment. It made me envious.

I was somewhat transfixed by the picture when the doc made his entry. I have known Dr. Freudenburg for quite some time. I taught his daughter college preparatory chemistry. He is a big man with a terrific bedside manner. I always get a kick out of his hair. The doc clearly has matters more important to attend to than combing his hair.

After shaking hands and exchanging greetings, he asked, "So, what's goin' on?" In answering, I largely repeated what I had told the nurse. I suspect Doc was reading her notes because as I spoke he was looking into my folder. As I spoke and he read, the doc commented, "Uh-uh, uh-uh," several times. We both finished at about the same time.

"Let's have a look at you," he said as he directed me to stand. He used his thumb to tug at the tops of my cheeks, exposing the portions of my eyeballs normally concealed by my lower eyelids. "You look anemic," he commented. I later came to the conclusion that he made the diagnosis of anemia as soon as he walked through the door and got his first look at me. "Let's have you jump up on the table," were his next words. He took a look into my ears and down my throat. Next, he used the stethoscope around my torso as I either took deep breaths or breathed normally.

The next part of the exam had me back on my feet. I had to bare my butt. The doc apologetically explained he needed a stool sample to test for the presence of blood. The sample he extracted was miniscule and, judging from Doc's comments, marginal. He had it tested anyway. The result was negative. Good. Maybe. What if the smallness of the sample rendered an inaccurate result? If another sample would be necessary, I hoped I could provide it the easy way by bringing it to the office the next morning.

Again, in retrospect I think he had already determined that I was anemic, so he was still looking for the cause, I am sure, when he said, "I want you to get some chest x-rays and then bring them right back over here." Off I went to the clinic's radiology department, which was about a forty-second walk away.

Within fifteen minutes, I was back in another one of the doc's examination rooms with my x-rays in hand. He seemed a little slow in getting to me this time, but I again noted that the place was very busy. So, I waited patiently.

Perhaps after a wait of about ten minutes, in came the doc. He apologized for the delay and thanked me for my patience. I sincerely assured him I understood that he was a busy man. Upon spying the over-sized envelope, he took the x-rays and put them up on the viewing screen. Almost immediately, he announced that they looked good. "I can't see any sign of cancer," he commented as he continued to examine the pictures. "I'll have a radiologist look these over, but he won't find anything," were his last words regarding the x-rays as he pivoted to look in my direction.

The doc's mention of cancer had no effect on me. Of course I did not have cancer.

The cause of my anemia was still unknown.

In his pursuit of an explanation for my anemia, which he still had not officially diagnosed, Dr. Freudenburg had me go to have blood drawn. This, too, would be done in the clinic. After the blood was drawn, Doc told me to go home and to expect a call from his office by no later than twelve-thirty that day. I was to stick by the phone. He also advised me that if the blood work showed normal, his nurse would call. If it was not normal, he would call, but I was not to panic at hearing his voice on the phone. "Hmmm," I thought, and replied that I would be waiting for a call.

I returned home to have some lunch. Eva had brought home

some wonderful sandwiches made by the deli department of a local butcher shop. While we ate our sandwiches, I related to her all that had gone on at the clinic. I was hungry, so my sandwich disappeared rather quickly. On the other hand, half of Eva's sandwich was clearly destined for the refrigerator. I considered eating the remaining half of Eva's sandwich, and she would have surely given it to me. I decided not. I later wished I had. My lunch would be the last real meal I would have to eat for the next nine days.

A little past noon, the phone rang. I answered to hear, "Hello, Jim. This is Dr. Freudenburg." I knew as per our previous discussion that the sound of his voice meant there was something wrong with my blood.

"Hi, Doc. What's up?" I replied.

As it turned out, it was not a matter of what was up. It was a matter of what was down. The doc informed me that my hemoglobin count had plummeted. In October of '06, when I was in for my annual physical, the count had been 15.6. Today, April 5, '07, the count was 7.2. Doc was right all along. Now the reason behind my loss of blood had to be determined.

The conversation concluded with Dr. Freudenburg informing me that I had an appointment with Dr. Philip Coff, a gastrointestinal specialist, at two o'clock that afternoon. Dr. Freudenburg had made the appointment for me. Dr. Freudenburg was so concerned with my condition that he asked Dr. Coff, as a professional courtesy, to squeeze me into his appointment schedule that afternoon. I thanked Dr. Freudenburg for his concern, and I assured him that I would be at Dr. Coff's office at the appointed time. I hung up the phone and turned to Eva, who had been listening all along.

My wife is a smart woman, and she did not like the sound of things. She informed me that she was taking the rest of the day off from work and that she would accompany me to my appointment with Dr. Coff. Shortly past one-thirty, I was headed to the clinic once again. Eva drove.

For the second time that day, I checked into the clinic. With paperwork in hand, Eva and I proceeded to Dr. Coff's office. After a very minimal wait in the lobby, we found ourselves seated in one of the doctor's examination rooms. As expected, a nurse was soon with us to take my vitals and other relevant information. When finished, the nurse left. Eva and I awaited the doctor, both of us anxious about my developing situation. My guess was that Eva was more worried than me. She did, after all, take the rest of the day off to be with me. I, on the other hand, was still confident that I would be leaving the doc's office with a prescription, a modified diet and orders for rest. Eva's instincts in these matters are always better than mine.

Without any warning, the door opened and Dr. Coff popped in. He is very much different in appearance than Dr. Freudenburg. He is close to my height and weight: five six and about one sixty-five. He and I have about the same amount of hair, which is to say practically none. Dr. Freudenburg would have been the perfect subject for a medical scene painted by Norman Rockwell. Dr. Coff looked like a medical professor at an Austrian university, circa late nineteenth and early twentieth centuries. He not only looked like such a professor to me, he had the mannerisms I would associate with such a person, too. I got the impression that the man is very competent and serious about his business. I understood why Dr. Freudenburg wanted me to see this guy.

Of course, Dr. Coff asked about my symptoms. I repeated them yet again. He wanted to know if I had experienced any abdominal pain or loss of weight or blood in my stool. "No," was my reply to all of these symptoms. I think he also asked me something about waking up in the night feeling sweaty, but I cannot recall exactly how he phrased his inquiry. In any event, I had had no "night time" troubles worth reporting, in my opinion.

Next, I went to the examination table. A stethoscope once again traveled around my torso. I cannot recall if Dr. Freudenburg did what followed, but if he did, he did not do so to the extent Dr. Coff would. As one might expect a GI doctor to do, Dr. Coff used his hands and fingers to extensively probe around my abdomen, always asking if I felt pain as he pushed and poked. I always answered that I felt no pain.

The exam was over. I adjusted my shirt and pants, and then I sat in the chair next to Eva's. The doc took a minute to add to the notes he started at the beginning of the session. After concluding his notations, Dr. Coff swiveled on his stool such that he was facing us. At the doc's request, I restated the symptoms I had been experiencing. He listened thoughtfully. When I finished, he once again asked if I had undergone any of the symptoms he queried about earlier. As before, I answered in the negative. I then followed with a few questions of my own regarding vigorous exercise, pushing a lawnmower and the like. As he gently shook his head in answer to my questions, Dr. Coff had a look on his face that struck me as being at the same time incredulous and sympathetic. Looking back on the moment, I would guess that he was thinking something to the effect, "This guy doesn't get it. He's not even going home today."

"I want you to check into the hospital," were the doc's next words to me, followed by, "You are not to go home to pick up a toothbrush or reading material or anything. Your wife can get any such items for you later." The hospital to which the doctor referred was Longmont United Hospital (LUH).

Eva and I exchanged looks, saying nothing.

He went on to warn that my condition was very serious, and that it was absolutely necessary to find out how it was that I had lost so much blood. The doc informed us that I would be getting a blood transfusion immediately upon my being hospitalized. Blood transfusion? I did not like the sound of "blood transfusion." I liked my own blood, but apparently I did not have much left. Furthermore, I recalled trouble with tainted blood years earlier. I supposed that that sort of trouble with the blood supply had been largely eradicated through improved screening techniques. I concluded that the odds were in my favor. The concept of probability would soon have a very *medically* significant role in my life.

Dr. Coff's last remark was, "I'll have a room reserved for you before you check in."

Before I checked in? Impressive. The hospital was only across the street.

The three of us stood, and I shook the doc's hand as Eva and I expressed our thanks. We opened the door, left the room and headed for the elevator. I am confident in stating that things had taken a turn that neither Eva nor I had anticipated. Heck, I would not have even gone to see a doctor that day had it not been for Eva's urging. I commented that "this" was clearly not on the spring break to-do list. Eva concurred.

Most of the rest or our conversation on the way to the hospital concerned how we would have to handle the logistics of my being there. Our main worry was about Boots. Her sitter, "Auntie K," would be out of town for the next six weeks. The hospital's being close to our home would help to mitigate Auntie's absence. I hoped for a short stay in the hospital, further mitigating Auntie's absence. My hope would be short-lived.

CHAPTER THREE

Welcome to the Hotel NoFoodForYa'

ITHIN THE SPAN of minutes, Eva and I had left the clinic's parking lot, crossed over Mountain View Avenue and were seeking a space in Longmont United Hospital's patients' parking lot. As we left the car, Eva told me to relax; she would attend to the preliminary details of my incarceration or, in other words, checking me into the hospital. She was trying to minimize my stress, and I appreciated her concern.

Dr. Coff had been true to his word. There was a room awaiting me, and with surprising efficiency, I was bound for it. In spite of this efficiency, I was less than pleased with having to be wheeled in a wheelchair to my room, as per hospital policy. I felt humiliated sitting in that chair, whose locomotion was provided by an elderly volunteer. I certainly had nothing against the volunteer. It was more that my being seated in a wheel chair implied that I needed help. The problem was, I *did* need help. I had not been able to figure out and cure my problem on my own. I abhor having to depend on others. In the days ahead, I would grudgingly have to accept being dependent upon others to an even greater extent, much greater.

By the time I was wheeled into my new quarters, room 4006, I had collected a small entourage of medical staff. It consisted of two RN's, one CNA and an admission person. They were all female. The male volunteer who wheeled me to my room left immediately upon my being seated on the bed. Lucky dog.

I felt like I was a queen, strictly in the sense of the word as it applies to a bee or ant colony. Clearly, I was my entourage's singular purpose. The fifth woman in the room was, of course, Eva. My wife is a person who truly puts the needs of others ahead of her own, and people are quick to sense this quality about her. I have contended for years that the joy she takes in helping others is one big reason she has been successful in business, and she has been very successful. My needs are always first among her priorities.

As each of the medical staff performed her duties, Eva floated around the perimeter of my bed performing her own assumed duties. She stored the street clothes that I had to remove, started a running list of things she would bring from home, helped provide personal medical information requested of me and adjusted my bed, bedding and gown to promote my comfort. Not only was Eva making note of what was being said and done, but also of what was left unsaid and undone.

After recording the necessary information about me, the admission lady closed her laptop and was the first staff member to leave my room. The CNA followed soon thereafter. When it appeared the

RN's were about to part company with me, satisfied that they were finished with their duties, Eva asked, "Where's the blood?"

"Blood?" the nurses replied.

"Yeah," Eva said. "The doctor said Jim was to start getting blood right away."

It is probable that I would have failed to mention this not-so-little detail to the nurses. I tend to overlook such things, but not my wife. Now, it is not my intention to suggest that the blood would never have gotten to me, only that Eva saw to it that the blood was gotten to me sooner than later.

By the time the last of my medical entourage left, I lay in the bed hooked up to an IV system. The IV needle ended up being in my right arm because two attempts to find a suitable vein in my left arm ended in failure. I wondered if the nurses' difficulty in finding a suitable vein was due to my severe anemia. Anyway, all's well that ends well. The IV needle was now allowing for two different liquids to enter my body. One liquid was a clear solution that served a nutritional function. The other liquid was blood, my most pressing concern.

When the first unit of blood arrived, I was impressed with the procedure that the nurses followed as a means of protecting the patient. Before the blood IV is started, the information on the blood bag is read aloud by one nurse as another nurse checks that the information being read matches the information on the patient's data sheet. Since this check is performed in the presence of the patient, he or she could act as an unofficial participant in this procedure. In my case, however, I would have been able to verify information such as my name and date of birth, but not my blood type. I learned that my blood type is AB positive by listening to the nurses crosschecking my personal information. I probably knew my blood type at some point in the past, but had long since forgotten it. If I could have chosen the type of blood I wanted, I would have chosen type S, as in Superman blood. I wanted an easy fix and a quick exit from the hospital. I was dreaming.

I would also end up dreaming of food during the course of my stay at LUH. I did not know it at the time, but my diet had become describable in two words: clear liquids. Furthermore, its description would ultimately deteriorate to two worse words: ice chips. To use the word loosely, very loosely, anything to do with cuisine, insofar as I was the subject, was contained in the ever-present IV bag. I appreciate that the contents of this bag helped to sustain me. But said contents could never satisfy my desire to eat, as in chew and swallow food, such as pizza.

Some several days into my hospitalization, a nurse attempted to season my Spartan cuisine with some humor. She joked that she sometimes liked to refer to a spent IV bag and its replacement in terms of menu entrees. For instance, she might say of the spent bag, "Oh, Mr. Gaudio, I see you've finished your steak and potatoes." Then of the replacement, she could follow up with something like, "Let's give you a little lasagna next." My response to the nurse's attempt at humor was a weak grin and a slight nod, without comment. I understood that the nurse was only trying to make a difficult circumstance a little less painful, and I certainly did not wish to hurt her feelings. But I was not in the mood for humor at that point, especially concerning food. In fact, at that time it was impossible for me to imagine that when I would be days deeper into this forced fast, I would find myself *un*interested in food.

From Thursday through Sunday, I would ultimately receive five units of blood: three on Thursday, one on Friday and one on Saturday. I think eight to ten units constitute a complete oil change. A unit is about a pint. I did wonder on several occasions whose blood was benefiting me. It became my intention to repay the blood I had taken from the supply. In fact, I came to feel guilty about not having given blood in the past when there were opportunities for me to do so. Laziness and, to a greater extent, an intense dislike of needles left me delinquent in this societal duty. My performance of this duty would simply have to improve in the future.

Eva, among others, started to comment about my improved color after I had gotten three units of blood. Truthfully, when I looked at a mirror I could not see much, if any, change in my complexion. As we talked about my newly acquired blush, Eva expressed some guilt over not noticing my paleness as it developed over the prior weeks. There was no need to feel guilty or embarrassed, in my opinion, and I told her so. I think it is easy to overlook gradual changes in someone with whom you live and see every day. What I mostly noticed as being a benefit from the boost in my blood supply was the disappearance of what I had come to call "my jumpy legs." I had developed so much involuntary jumpiness in my legs, especially at night, I wondered if I had restless leg syndrome.

In our first moment alone in my room, Eva and I could talk of nothing but our disappointment over my current predicament. It was also probable that Eva was concerned about my reaction to all of this. Knowing me as she does, there would have been ample reason to expect me to be difficult in this situation. However, I would come to surprise, if not shock, both of us through this ordeal. With the exception of one minor episode, I maintained an attitude of resignation to the point of docility throughout my stay in the hospital. I figured what the heck else could I do? Clearly I was sick, and this was the only way to figure out what was wrong and to develop a medical response. Also, this tumult had to be very nerve wracking for Eva. There was no point in my making her even more upset.

Around five o'clock, Eva left for home to get the things we thought necessary for my stay in the hospital. Not long after she had gone, Dr. Coff stopped in to see me. He looked things over, including me, and seemed satisfied that all was proceeding as he expected. The doc then informed me that, pursuant to the mission of determining what was causing my blood loss, I would be undergoing an endoscopy and colonoscopy early on Friday. This meant no food for me and that I would have to completely evacuate my bowels. In departing, he assured me that the solution that would induce the evacuation would be delivered forthcoming, and that I was to have it all downed by nine o'clock. My first encounter with the aforementioned solution (or its equivalent) occurred some years earlier. I remembered the encounter only too well. I was in for a miserable night.

I must mention, for the record, that I was not worried about the colonoscopy, itself. I did this gig once before because my primary care physician at the time said it is the thing to start doing, every five years or so, once one reaches fifty years of age. As I endured this medical procedure six years earlier, I almost pulled whatever was rammed up my butt, out. Had I done so, I would have terminated the session when I was about half way through it. I was tempted in this fashion because I was in excruciating pain and very angry because of it. The only reason I did not abort the procedure was because of all the prior torture I had endured in emptying my bowels as preparation. I swore at the time that I would never, as in *never*, endure a colonoscopy again. The reason that I was so relaxed about undergoing another such examination the next day was because when Dr. Freudenburg became my family physician, he told me that a colonoscopy does not have to be painful. He was appalled at my earlier experience, calling it "barbaric." I concurred. Doc assured me that there are drugs that make this exam a nonevent. This knowledge made me unconcerned with the morrow. The four liters of the bowel evacuating solution, GoLYTELY (brand name), to be downed in fewer than four hours was another matter.

By the time Eva returned to the hospital, I had begun drinking the GoLYTELY. It tasted as obnoxious as I had remembered. When I swallow this solution, it leaves a residual scent in my nasal passages. It is almost as if I can simultaneously smell and taste it, a terrible one-two punch. I really hate this stuff. I tried to combat the aftertaste by chasing the solution with a swig or two of cranberry juice. The juice serves as a masking agent. A masking agent is no help, however, in dealing with the matter of volume. Four liters is a little more than a gallon. This is a daunting amount, even if one were dealing with a palatable beverage, like beer. I cannot imagine that even the Cone-heads would want to "consume mass quantities" of GoLYTELY. If they had, they would be spending mass amounts of time on the toilet. Once the first urge to visit the commode is induced, one best stay close, very close, to the bathroom. At the point at which I had drunk about a third of the total, there was no appreciable lag between downing a cup and the need to have my butt on the commode. And there is no doubt as to whether the sensation one feels is gas or not. It is not! By this point of the ordeal, I was thinking a more suitable name for this laxative would be Go-*NOT*-so-lytely. This whole purging experience can be summed up in one word: Crappy.

I am always amazed at how freely we talk to our medical caregivers about personal matters when in a medical facility. Pooping is not typically a subject of normal social discourse. Yet when one is a patient in a hospital, not only is pooping a probable subject of prominent interest, but the details of an episode of this biological function might be rather graphic. Details related to pooping would dominate my first night in the hospital, such as: Did I poop? How much did I poop? Am I still pooping? What's the poop look like? And, of course the most important pooping question of all: Am I finally done pooping?

As strange as it may sound, I was glad Eva was present to help me in performing a duty I usually prefer to perform in private. Once she returned from home, I was able to quickly get her up to speed. When the action inevitably began, she assisted me in every way that she could. For instance, wherever I went, the IV tree, as I came to call it, was sure to follow. Eva guided the tree to and from the bathroom, relieving me of the trouble. She also played bartender, continually bringing me cups of laxative solution to drink, followed by cups of cranberry juice. Anything she could do to make an uncomfortable situation more comfortable, she gladly and lovingly did.

There were, of course, some things she could not help me through. As an example, even though she could get the IV tree to and from the bathroom for me, the IV line itself was a problem for me when I was on the commode. As mentioned previously, the IV needle was stuck in my right arm, and I am right handed. This meant that cleaning myself had to be done with my left hand. By the time the laxative had run its course, I was rather impressed with the degree of ambidexterity I had developed in this matter. Speaking of cleaning, I have some advice for those who find themselves in my situation. The need to clean during one of these sessions is frequent. The anal orifice will take a frictional pounding from the frequent use of dry toilet paper. So, have plenty of moistened wipes present to minimize the irritation.

Suffice it to say that the ordeal extended until after midnight, even though I had downed the last of the laxative by nine o'clock. When all gastrointestinal sensations had ceased, I knew I was finally empty. Eva had decided she was staying over night. She settled into her pullout bed and we both went to sleep. I was exhausted, so I slept quite well. I think Eva slept reasonably well, too. The troublemaker within me did not sleep a wink, however.

CHAPTER FOUR

The C-Word Lurks

WE WERE BOTH up by six o'clock the next morning. I am sure that Eva must have had something for breakfast, but I cannot recall exactly what it was. I was too selfishly consumed by my silent complaint that I was not allowed to break *my* fast. Anyway, my attention would soon be diverted from food. At about eight o'clock, two hospital staff members showed up to transfer me to the room where the endoscopy and colonoscopy would be performed. "Terrific," I thought. "Let's get this done, and I'll have a good meal afterward."

The two ladies who wheeled me along on my gurney were of good humor that morning. One pushed and the other guided, as we joked and laughed about various things along the route. Eva, of course, made the trip with me, and she was being her usual bright and cheerful self. This would be the last time we would be in such light spirits, though, for some days ahead.

When we arrived at our destination, in no more than five minutes travel time, Dr. Coff had yet to arrive. The two attending nurses knew what the game plan was, so they began to prepare for the procedures, at least as far as they could in the doc's absence. One of the two nurses was particularly chatty. At one point in our wait for Dr. Coff, she volunteered that I would breeze right through my examinations because I would have had the "I don't care about anything" drug in advance. Good. This was in line with what Dr. Freudenburg had mentioned that day in his office. I was all the more eager to get the procedures started and done. "And let's hope this bleeding you're having is just a matter of a simple ulcer that can be easily corrected," the same nurse encouraged. I had not thought about an ulcer. I did not like considering that having to deal with an ulcer would likely necessitate an undesirable change in my diet, at least temporarily. Yet, my limited medical knowledge suggested that an ulcer should be something modern medical science could easily correct. At this point, I would have gladly settled for an ulcer as being the culprit, and gotten on with my life. Yes, an ulcer might have qualified as the easy and quick fix I was looking for.

Dr. Coff was about thirty minutes late from a procedure he did ahead of mine. His tardiness did not bother me. I understand that this medical stuff is not an exact science and that there are complications that can arise, playing havoc with a doctor's schedule. What was particularly note worthy to me, however, was that Dr. Freudenburg was with Dr. Coff. This surprised me. I considered this particularly caring on Dr. Freudenburg's part, and he is a caring man, to be sure. I would find out later that he had an ulterior motive for attending.

Well, once the doc showed up, things really got rolling. Eva departed for the waiting room, and the final stages of my preparation were completed. As I mentioned earlier, Dr. Coff is all business. I last remember being told to roll onto my left side. I remember nothing of the procedures, nor do I remember anything of the return trip to my room. The first thing I remember is realizing that I was back in my bed in room 4006. Had I not been told the procedures were performed, I would have had no idea that they had been. There was no evidence that I could feel that instruments had been run down my throat or up my butt. My experience was anything but barbaric, but what were the results?

We had not been in my room for too long before Dr. Coff showed up. Without ado, he informed me that the endoscopy and colonoscopy did not reveal my problem. Drat. I tried to look on the bright side of things. At least the colonoscopy did not reveal that I had colorectal cancer. And I *did* treat this as good news, as Dr. Freudenburg must have, too. I would ultimately learn that Dr. Freudenburg attended the colonoscopy because he was of the opinion that my anemia was caused by colon cancer. For that matter, Dr. Coff may have been of the same opinion. In any event, the mystery continued, and I do not like mysteries, especially when they concern my deteriorating health. I was losing hope that my problem would be fixed easily and quickly.

Up next was a CAT-scan, as per Dr. Coff's orders. He told me that I would be going for the scan as soon as I could be fit into the scanner's schedule. His order for this exam dashed my plan for a well-deserved meal. The closest I would get to anything like a milkshake was a barium-containing "solution," about a quart of it. As with the laxative, the barium solution showed up as promised. Its consumption was also timed. I think that I had to have it all down in twenty minutes.

Eva had intended to accompany me to this exam, too, but she missed it. Since we live so close to the hospital, we gambled that she could quickly run home to check on things, particularly the dog, and make it back in time for my CAT-scan. Wrong. Not long after she had left for home, a guy working as what used to be called an orderly showed up with a wheelchair. In a jiffy, I found myself seated in the chair and bound for the CAT-scan department.

I was glad that a CAT-scan is not like an MRI. Instead of being placed into a very confining tube, a CAT-scan simply requires the patient to be passed through a ring-type structure, while lying down. I dubbed the ring structure "the portal," because it reminded me of something form an old episode of Star Trek. When lying down, the patient is on a conveyor. It is the conveyor that moves the patient back-and-forth through the portal in a manner necessary to perform the patient's examination.

Being CAT-scanned is fast and easy. My exam was done in a matter of minutes. Before I knew it, I was back in the wheelchair and on my way to my room, with the help of the same orderly. Eva was waiting for me when I arrived, a mite disappointed that she was not present to accompany me to the scan room. She takes her duties as my guardian angel very seriously, for which I am eternally grateful. After Eva was satisfied that I somehow managed to survive in her absence, she allowed my inquiries about how things looked at home. I was especially interested to know how Boots soloed (her first) overnight. It comforted me to learn that all was well and good on the home front, including our beloved Boots. We were talking about this little dog of ours when Dr. Coff made a purposeful entry into my room.

"I didn't expect to see you so soon, Doc. What's up?" I asked.

"The CAT-scan shows you have a tumor in your small intestine," he answered, while looking me squarely in the eyes.

Hmmm. A tumor.

I had never even considered a tumor as a possibility, and I did not like the sound of this, not one iota. Eva and I reflexively glanced at one another at the instant the doc ended his sentence. Eva's face displayed a blend of shock and fear. Mine must have, too. It was beginning to feel like I could not catch a break. Like some gambler who had run afoul of Lady Luck, I was on a bad losing streak. Gamblers like to say that the only way to weather a streak of bad luck is to play through it. I figured I would roll the dice again by asking, "Is it cancerous?" I know that this was exactly the question on Eva's mind, and I figure it is a safe bet that the doc saw it coming.

"There's no way to tell from the scan," the doctor replied, with a tone of sympathy to his voice. Anticipating my next question, he quickly followed with, "The only way to know will require surgery."

Hmmm. Surgery.

Surgery was something else I had never considered upon admission to the hospital. I had my tonsils taken out in nineteen fifty-six or seven, and I underwent a hemorrhoidectomy in nineteen eighty-six. Over the years, I saw something of a wry humor to the oppositeness of the locations of these two procedures. Now I faced having to deal with something in between the extremities of my previous surgeries. And this something could very conceivably be life threatening.

"When, Doc?"

"If I can get the surgeon I want, Monday."

Hmmm. Monday.

I do not like to have to wait to find out about something that is personally important, such as the outcome of a job interview, let alone something that is possibly a matter of life or death. Unfortunately, wondering whether or not the tumor was malignant would be unavoidable for Eva and me over the next several days. This would be one of those times in life when I wished I had a crystal ball. And there is such a thing, sort of.

I have always found the mathematics of calculating probability to be fascinating. Although statistical probability is not the same thing as a magical crystal ball, such mathematics give us our best means by which to get a sense of the future likelihood of some event. Two masters of such mathematics are the insurance companies and the casino operators. They have applied their skills with probability mathematics incredibly profitably. Surely there had to be some malignancy probability in regards to my tumor. It seemed sensible to me that Dr. Coff's experience should allow him to make a reasonable prognostication about my tumor being benign or malignant. I was very aware that I would be essentially asking the doctor to make an educated guess, and I also understood that probability does not equal certainty. But I was eager for a ray of hope in a future that suddenly looked bleak. Even a sixty-forty chance favoring "benign" would have provided us with some comfort. I pressed.

"Doc," I began, "can you give me some kind of feel for the chances of the tumor being malignant? Fifty-fifty? Better (for me)? Worse?"

I suspect Doc had been down this road quite some several times before my case. He gently shook his head back and forth before speaking, something like an adult would do as the front end of a response to a child's preposterous question. Even before he spoke, I knew that he was not going to pin himself to some statement of probability. "No. I can't," broke his silence.

Maybe the doc's response meant that he could not, or maybe it meant that he would not. At the time, I did not know. During a subsequent conversation with my surgeon, I realized, in retrospect, that Dr. Coff *would not*, and for good reason.

I pressed the doc no more. I would simply have to hunker down and await my fate, knowing that it would not allow for a fast and easy fix.

The way that I see it, the first CAT-scan was like a military reconnaissance flight that located the enemy. The enemy's position, once known, had to be better defined in order to promote the development of the most effective attack against it. This is the reason Dr. Coff told me that I would be immediately prepared for a follow-up scan. The surgeon would want to be as familiar with my body's invader as possible. In short order, four pints of what I presume to be various versions of barium solution showed up at my room. The scan technician, whom I recognized from my first scan, delivered them, herself. I was to drink one of the four within the first twenty minutes of their delivery. When the first twenty-minute period expired, I was to drink a second pint within the second twenty-minute period. When the second twenty-minute period expired, I was to continue with the last two pints as I had with the first two. The barium concoctions, all five, were not as bad as the GoLYTELY, but I am certain that they represent no threat to taking a share of the "smoothies" market. The only person who felt worse than I about my having to guzzle these various solutions over the last eighteen hours was Eva. It is her way to put others ahead of herself.

I followed the technician's instructions to the letter. I had already made up my mind that I was going to give every medical person connected to my treatment all the help that I could provide. The only thing that was in my direct control was the degree of cooperation I could provide in my care. I would dot all the i's and cross all the t's. Period.

The second CAT-scan was a bit lengthier and required more of me in terms of breathing and holding my breath upon command, but it was essentially as easy as the first. Also, before I was allowed to return to my room, some higher-up person had to read the scans. When this person was satisfied that the scans were of sufficient detail, back to room 4006 I went, with Eva at my side. She had waited for me in the hallway because the patient is the only person allowed in the scan area during the procedure. Even the operating technician was within a glass-walled control room as she operated the scanner.

At this point, Eva and I were reconciled to my situation. My reconciliation took the form of a resolve to cooperate to my utmost, as previously mentioned. Eva's took the form of assisting me in every way she possibly could. Over the coming days, the only way Eva could have spent more time in the hospital would have been if she had been an in-patient herself. Such a display of spousal dedication, if I may say so myself, and I will, would be quite some feat by anyone. In my wife's case it was made all the more impressive due to her position of president and CEO of a mid-size credit union. I realize that the title CEO often conjures up negative images of some overpaid fat cat who is insulated by multiple layers of subordinates. My wife is the antithesis of this description. Nothing could prove this more than the fact that her office is directly off the main lobby, and it is not shielded by a receptionist or secretary. Credit union members often saunter uninvited into my wife's office, confident of receiving a warm reception and sincere attentiveness. Even though the interloper should have taken his or her concern to someone in a department specifically designed to deal with it, my wife will disrupt her schedule to help resolve the member's concern, even if it borders being trivial.

Although the admission pains me, the truth is I had become a disruption to my wife's work schedule, but she did not even flinch. In the complete absence of any fluster, Eva immediately resolved to scale back her schedule to skeletal status. And believe me, even in skeletal form, her schedule would cause most equivalent professionals to plummet into a state of hopeless despair. We understood that I was going to be in the hospital for probably more than a week. So Eva, being the problem-solving type, decided she would set up a crude office in my room. I was amazed at how efficiently this can be done, using the modern technological wonders of a laptop computer (with wifi access) and a cell phone. I, too, would come to directly benefit from her makeshift office. While operating mostly from this off-site office, Eva communicated with the top-notch staff she had assembled over the years to keep the credit union operating on a business-as-usual basis. True to her character, my wife would give most of the credit for this accomplishment to her staff and a very sympathetic board of directors. But I will say without reservation that my wife juggled home, profession and cancer patient husband like nobody else can.

As for my part in all of this, I very much appreciated that Eva wanted to attend to me, first and foremost. Equally, however, I also understood that the world does not stop just because Jim Gaudio is in the hospital. The fact was that Eva had professional duties and responsibilities that only she, herself, could address. It was my hope that Eva's being able to keep tabs on the credit union would help to make her stressful situation less so. I was also hopeful that Eva's being able to do some work would serve as a constructive distraction for her. In looking back, I think that both my hopes were met.

At the time Dr. Coff entered my room, Eva and I were ironing out the details of the adjustments we would be making in our life over the coming days. With his usual business-like demeanor, the doctor informed us that the details provided by the second CAT-scan were satisfactory. He seemed confident in stating that my tumor was about the size of a tennis ball and that it was located about midway along the small intestine. I was more impressed by the thing's girth than its address along my small bowel. Based upon the date of my last annual checkup, I figured the tumor had achieved its size in about five months.

From the moment that I knew I had an operable tumor, I intuitively understood that the surgeon would become the pivotal actor in my little drama. I was eager to meet this surgeon, one Dr. Coff clearly held in high regard. The doctor advised me to expect the surgeon to stop by to examine me at his earliest convenience. After receiving this information, we thanked the doc yet again, and then he left. Now alone in my room, Eva and I resumed our attempt to adjust ourselves to our reordered life. I suppose such adjustments are ongoing in life, but at some times much more conspicuously than at others.

Dr. John Leonard entered room 4006 much like a gust of wind blasts into a room through an open window. That is, he was suddenly present, and his presence claimed one's attention as its just due. He was wearing much of a surgeon's outfit, even the cap. I liked the cap. I still want to get one for myself. The garb made any need to make reference to his specialty superfluous. After a quick introduction of himself, he strode with deliberation toward an unoccupied chair near the foot of my bed. At reaching his destination, he heavily dropped himself into the chair, revealing that he had long been on his feet, likely in surgery.

He looked familiar.

With an amused look, he inquired, "Are you the chemistry teacher at Skyline?"

"Ah, yes. He's Dr. *Leonard*, Leonard as in Megan Leonard, a former chemistry student of mine," I mentally stated. It had probably been eight or ten years since I talked to the doctor at parent-teacher conferences. But the more I studied his face and the manner in which he sat, I could imagine seeing him seated across the table from me all those years ago.

He would have had more trouble recognizing me than my name. Since I had last seen the doc I changed my appearance. I now wore only a mustache, instead of a full beard. Furthermore, I came to keep what hair I have left cut extremely short, just a notch above being shaved.

With a broad smile I replied, "Yes, I am."

"I thought it had to be you. There aren't many Gaudios around these parts, you know," he accurately observed.

What a coincidence. Two of my three doctors were the fathers of girls who were former chemistry students of mine. I was pleased to be able to recall that I had had a good rapport and relationship with Dr. Leonard over the span of his daughter's studies with me. I do not know how I would have felt had he been some parent with whom I had been at odds over his child's performance in my class. Hey, I already had enough "bad blood" going for me.

Of course, the doctor already knew what my situation was, and he spoke to me about it frankly and honestly, man-to-man. While explaining what was going on inside me and what was to be done about it, the doc would vacillate between using language that was technical and colloquial. For instance, he used Latin sounding terms to describe the tumor's location, but he chose to describe the quality of my blood as being diluted wine. This range of language was consistent with the range of his personality, as I would learn over the days ahead.

After giving me the down and dirty of my circumstance, Dr. Leonard wanted to examine me. His examination was purely manual, poking and pushing his way around the area of my lower intestine. He was trying to feel for the tumor. He said it was difficult to locate by feeling for it, and would probably miss it if he did not know it was there in the first place. Nonetheless, the exam led him to speculate that the tumor could be about the size of his fist. The doc is a big man with large, thick hands. His estimate of size was considerably greater than that of Dr. Coff's. I did not like how my tumor seemed to be growing.

At this point I knew that I had a tumor; it was located in my small intestine; its size was substantial; and I was bleeding internally through it.

I still did not know if it was benign or malignant, however.

"What do you think, Doc, malignant or benign?" I ventured.

Like Dr. Coff, Dr. Leonard would not guess.

"Guessing is too risky," was Dr. Leonard's deflective response.

He went on to explain that guessing in a situation such as mine is bad medical practice. If the guess, right or wrong, goes in the patient's favor, it is euphoria. If the opposite occurs, it is the pits. I appreciated the doctor's position, and I now also understood why it was that Dr. Coff refused to offer a guess earlier. Only time, itself, could reveal what I wanted to know. At this point, I decided to expect the tumor to be malignant. I thought this to be prudent because nobody was telling me something to the effect of, "Don't worry about the tumor. We see this kind all the time. They're always benign." If it turned out benign, terrific, if not, I would have prepared for the worst. I said nothing of my decision to Eva.

Next, the doctor talked to me about some of the particulars of my surgery. He told me that a less invasive procedure (laparoscopy) was not an option in my case. It was necessary that I would have a large incision, probably six or seven inches in length, minimum.

This was no big deal to me; my Speedo swimwear days were long behind me. The doc also warned me that there would be a lot of pain with this surgery. Pain always gets my attention. Nobody has ever had justification to think me masochistic. I was relieved when Doc followed up by assuring me that medical science had gotten a lot better over the last thirty-some years at helping patients deal with pain. It was better still to learn that he was going to provide me with the Cadillac (his description) of pain management systems. This system would consist of two components: a pain ball pumping painkilling medicine into the area all around the incision, and an epidural. I had never heard of a pain ball, but I had of an epidural, as used to assist women in labor. It sounded like the doc had designed a one-two punch to knock out my pain, and I was already appreciative of his efforts. Furthermore, I was by now feeling very confident in this guy's abilities. He was kind of cocky, but not to the great extent that his time-tested competence would have justified. And he let me know right from the start that my surgery would not be his "maiden voyage," that he had in fact been in the business of slicing people open for thirty-seven years. No, he allowed himself to be cocky just enough to encourage his patient's confidence in his surgical abilities. It was his way of telling the patient, "Lean on me; I can hold you up." Dr. Leonard understood both the physical and psychological dimensions of surgery. Dr. Coff had picked a good surgeon for me, a very good surgeon. And a good surgeon could be the ticket to a good conclusion to my troubles. Maybe things were starting to look up.

Before parting, the doc asked if I had any questions.

I had one: "When can I go back to work?"

"You're not," the doc shot back. "You're done for the year," he followed with a tone that was the blend of matter-of-factness and finality.

That was that.

The doc then informed me to expect him to stop by some time on Saturday. His purpose would be to impart some of the details of the game plan for Sunday, which would be the preparation day for my surgery on Monday. When he was satisfied that I was sufficiently informed, he was off, leaving Eva and me in the wake of his high-speed exit. We were both somewhat bewildered in the "Who-was-that-masked-man?" sort of way. In the coming days, we would learn that Dr. Leonard's visits are always an event.

Whether or not I made it to be fifty-seven or one hundred and seven, this Good Friday would serve as a high-water mark in my life. Eva and I limped through the rest of the day, doing this and that. We had decided that it would be best that she spend nights at home. For one thing, doing so would allow her a much better opportunity for a solid night's sleep. The pullout bed in my room was tolerable, but not as good as our bed. Just as significantly, getting a complete night's sleep in a hospital, in the absence of some form of sedation or sleep aide, is nigh impossible, as I was about to learn firsthand.

Although my wife is perfectly capable of taking care of herself, I insisted that she call me once she was safely installed in our home for the night. This became a matter of procedure during my stay at LUH.

Her first such call to me, however, stands out as the most memorable one. This is because Eva concluded the conversation by telling me, "Get a good night's sleep, now. Tomorrow, we go into battle mode." And we would do exactly that.

CHAPTER FIVE

Takin' Care of Business

FTER TURNING OFF my cell phone, Eva's words "battle mode" still resonated in my head. I looked at the clock and noted that midnight was just a few minutes into the future. Ah yes, the future, lying ahead shrouded in uncertainty.

I began to fret.

The truth be told, it was not my medical condition causing my worry. It was my students. I was going to have to abandon them. This would necessitate two events: the first would be an explanation from me to my students; the second would be their transition to someone who would serve as their new teacher for the remainder of the school year, about seven weeks. My head began to whir with the details of these matters of explanation and transition. Complicating things was my need to get all that needed doing done on Saturday because Sunday would find me medically preoccupied. I started to feel overwhelmed. My little world was collapsing around me. How would I deal with my suddenly very messy life?

It took several minutes, the clock now indicated a brand new day, but I got a grip on myself. In so doing I realized that the answer to my question was simple: I would deal with matters one at a time, taking the most important one first and then moving to the next most important and so on. I would approach what lay ahead to do on Saturday much like I would go about cleaning up a room victimized by entropy. And the best way to start this cleanup project, I concluded, was to get a good night's sleep. This would allow me to approach matters with clarity of mind and restored energy. As regards energy, I had better garner what I could from sleep because my diet was still limited to clear liquids. My guess was that once my guts had been purged, the intent was to keep them so.

I turned off the lights, and soon thereafter, fell into a sound sleep. This night's sleep would be one of the best, if not *the* best, I would get through my entire stay. I woke up at about five forty-five and ready to face the tasks of the day. I went into battle mode.

Eva would not arrive until about eight o'clock. While waiting for her, I hand wrote a letter to my students. Once the laptop arrived, I would enter the letter into the computer's memory and send it to my department chairman as an e-mail attachment. In the letter, I explained in minimal detail what had occurred and that my students and I would be severing ties, as a consequence. The letter was difficult to write for two reasons. Firstly, and to my considerable surprise, composing the letter was emotionally hard on me. A normal conclusion to a school year finds me, as it does most teachers, elated to be rid of my students, and I tell them this. I like to drive this point home during the last weeks of school by asking them the question, "Who's counting the days 'till the end of the school year even more than you students?" Invariably, they resoundly answer, "The teachers!" They're not stupid. Anyway, teachers and students parting company at the end of the school year is an event that is much anticipated and festive. *This* parting was anything but anticipated, and there was nothing festive about it. Secondly, it is my nature to be private, if not downright secretive, about matters of a personal nature. And I considered my medical condition to be deeply personal. Writing this letter to my students went against my grain. It is difficult for me to imagine another profession in which I would have felt compelled to write a letter similar to the one I wrote to my students.

My comments about my love of privacy might make it seem, at first, odd that I chose to have the letter I wrote to my students e-mailed to the entire staff at Skyline High. I figured what the heck. Once the cat was out of the bag, there was no sense in kidding myself that I still had some control over the cat because it had left some fur behind in the bag. The e-mail would also save various people from being inundated with questions about my absence.

Near the letter's end, I requested that people not visit or call me. The request, of course, was made in the interest of my privacy. Almost equally, however, this was my way of keeping the emotions of my situation under control, especially mine. It was my view that keeping the flow of people under control would work toward keeping the flow of emotions under control as well. I knew decades earlier that if I were to ever find myself in a situation like the one I was in, I would approach it in this reclusive way. My inspiration was a schoolmate from high school who died of testicular cancer when he was in his mid-twenties. He did likewise regarding visitations when in the hospital during his last days. By no means do I intend to suggest that I believed my situation to be legitimately comparable to his. I recognize that his policy fit my personality more than it did my situation, at least as far as I knew my situation to be.

The student letter follows.

April 9, 2007

Dear Students:

I will keep this brief.

Over spring break, I learned that I have a very serious medical problem. This problem will disallow my return to teaching for the remainder of the '06-'07 school year. I inform you of this matter with deep regret for various reasons. Also, please note that I will be of minimal help in your transition to a new teacher(s). This means that the smoothness of the transition process will be largely in your hands. I will, therefore, fully expect that you give your very best effort in solving all problems and in minimizing all difficulties related to my forced absence.

Finally, my inclination toward privacy and my need to apply my complete attention to my aforementioned medical problem, compel me to request that you do not attempt to call or visit me. Please understand that this request directs no rudeness toward you, nor does it seek to display any lack of appreciation for your concern for me. It is only that I must limit the emotion of my situation in order to keep it manageable. Know that I will make the same request of my colleagues.

So, life throws us another curve ball. Let's do our best to get good wood on it.

Most sincerely,

Mr. Gaudio

Eva showed up at the hospital at about eight o'clock. It was clear that a good night's sleep at home had produced the desired effect. She was refreshed and ready to tackle the day ahead. And a long day it was. Nonetheless, by day's end we had properly served notice of my need to take an extended leave from work, and we provided the information necessary to ease the impact of this imminent absence. I would have never made such productive use of the day without Eva's help. A cell phone and laptop, in conjunction with a terrific helpmate, allowed me to feel a sense of accomplishment at day's end. I was now satisfied that I could close the book on my professional responsibilities and focus on my medical needs.

There is something that should be mentioned about "closing the book" on my professional responsibilities on that Saturday. One project that was very important to complete on that day was my grade book, actually a computer program spread sheet. Getting the grade book current would provide valuable information to the kids' new teacher. In regards to the kids, the two courses I teach are as different as day and night in terms of student quality. My chemistry students are vastly superior students relative to my physical science kids. For instance, in updating the spreadsheets for the two sections of physical science, I had to make a tally of penalty deductions. Such deductions are incurred for failure to bring the textbook to class. Specifically, each time a physical science student fails to bring his or her textbook to class, I deduct five points from the kid's point total. This policy does not exist for my chemistry classes, for there is no need of it with my chemistry students. Anyhow, as I tallied up the penalties, I felt disgusted as I thought, "What a waste of my life. Here I am in the hospital with a tumor that I figure to be cancerous, and I'm tallying penalty points against students too lazy to bring their books to class." In that moment, I knew that I had to leave teaching in the public schools, and I had to leave soon, very soon.

As promised, Dr. Leonard came to visit me on Saturday. I had been correct in anticipating Sunday and Monday would be unavailable to use to wrap up my professional business for the school year. My schedule for Sunday would be dominated by preparation for surgery on Monday, although it was not possible to know an exact time on Monday at that point. Dr. Leonard explained that the surgery department operates on "its own time." Sometimes things in surgery go faster than expected, sometimes slower. I figured that I was being squeezed in and should be grateful for getting in at any time on Monday. Simply stated, I would go to surgery when the transport crew showed up to take me. Doc further informed me that the preparation regimen scheduled for Sunday would start with another session of GoLYTELY. I would begin drinking the four liters at eight o'clock, and the last drop had to be downed by noon. The intention of the second round of GoLYTELY was to make my guts super evacuated for surgery. My non-existent diet would assist the GoLYTELY in this purge. I had been, and would remain for the foreseeable future, on a clear liquid diet. The most substantial, using the word very loosely, food that appeared on my menu was a broth. I imagined it was some sort of beef or chicken broth made from bullion cubes. I never came to know for sure because I was not interested enough to ask. I figured what was the point in knowing what nothing was made from? The bottom line here is that the GoLYTELY would find little to resist it in my innards on Sunday.

Come the appointed time on Sunday, I got after the GoLYTELY in dogged fashion and had the container drained by ten thirty. The nurses working my room were amazed. It was their opinion that I had set a record.

My previous drinking bouts involving GoLYTELY, or its equivalent, left me plenty experienced regarding what I would be going through the next time around. It was the second part of the preparatory regimen that caught me off guard. Dr. Leonard wanted me purged, or nearly so, in another regard. When he had me opened up, it was the doctor's intention to look around. Part of this exploration would involve my colon. It would be prudent to reduce the bacteria population before handling this part of my anatomy. Pursuant to this objective, Dr. Leonard planned for me to take large doses of antibiotics on Sunday afternoon. He had prescribed three different antibiotics. I was to take a dose of each antibiotic at each session of dosing. The first session was scheduled for two o'clock, the second for three o'clock and the third for six o'clock. Each individual dose was one gram, so I would end up taking three grams of each antibiotic over the three dosing sessions.

Oftentimes, it is recommended that a dosage of a given drug be taken with a meal. I had not had anything that resembled what most folks in this country would consider a meal for over seventy-two hours when I began taking the prescribed antibiotics. In spite of my emptied stomach, I was optimistic that I could take all of these antibiotics with minimal undesirable side effects because I had never been particularly sensitive to medications. Of course, I failed to consider that I had never been dosed with any type of medication like I would be presently dosed with these antibiotics. Nevertheless, I tolerated the first batch of antibiotics well. At three o'clock, I was still feeling well when I downed the second batch. "So far, so good," I thought.

Even though it was Easter Sunday, our attorney and one of our closest of friends, Brian Holst, insisted on coming to the hospital to make sure that legal things like power of attorney were in order to his satisfaction. Brian is also a notary of the public, rendering the matter of legal signatures no problem. As Brian was explaining various legal matters pertinent to my surgery, I noticed that I was having difficulty focusing. In fact, an increasing feeling of nausea was distracting me. I had been sitting in a chair but decided I had better lie in bed. I explained to Eva that I thought the antibiotics were starting to make me ill. I hoped that I would not fall into feeling much worse than I did, but the six o'clock dosing session began to seriously worry me. Brian could see that I was starting to struggle, and he left so that I could privately cope with my new problem. My poor wife was once again forced to bear witness to my misery. I know that Eva' sense of empathy caused her heart to ache for me. She commenced to lovingly provide whatever assistance she could. If a sincere concern for my condition were able to cure me of all that was ailing me, Eva would have provided enough to have me on my feet and walking out of the hospital in a minute's time. But the only thing a minute's time brought me was one minute closer to six o'clock.

Indifferent to my plight, six o'clock arrived right on time, as always. The same nurse who had administered the first two dosing sessions delivered the third and final batch of my antibiotics. She was aware of my feeling ill, but the show had to go on, as per Dr. Leonard's orders. Again, I took each pill from its little condiment cup and then downed it with water. I had a bad feeling about this last batch, literally and figuratively. I braced myself for the worse.

By this point, I considered vomiting as being my main enemy. I did not want to render the doc's plans ineffective by throwing up the antibiotics before they had a chance to do their intended work. By eight o'clock, suppressing the feeling of needing to vomit was requiring a considerable amount of will power. I was hoping that the fact that there was so little in my stomach would allow me to hold out longer. Maintaining my resolve in this attempted suppression was getting harder and harder because I was getting sicker and sicker. I kept the puke pan perched on my chest as I sat up in bed, just in case. Eva kept applying folded washcloths moistened with cold water across my forehead to provide me with some relief. This went on until about ten thirty.

Seeing that Eva was exhausted, I told her that I wanted her to go home. Try as she may, there was really nothing she could do to minimize my plight. She packed up various items and bid me a very sad good night. Once home, she called me as per our safety-check routine. I hoped her exhaustion would overcome her concern about me and force her into a deep, restful sleep.

As for my getting any sleep, the nurse mentioned earlier that I was allowed to have an Ambien, if I so chose. It was now close to eleven, and I had managed to this point to avoid vomiting. I wondered if sleeping would allow me to avoid vomiting altogether. So, I rang for one of the nurses working the night shift and asked if I could please have an Ambien. Soon after my request, she had returned with the sleep aide. I chased it down the hatch with a few gulps of water. By this time, I had abandoned the little puke pan. Instead, I opted for a tub about the size necessary to soak one's feet. My thinking was, "The bigger the target, the better." It was a good decision. Not three minutes after taking the Ambien, I lost control of my ability to suppress the urge to vomit, and up it came. "It" was not much in terms of volume or mass. I would have called what I had expelled a bile, although I do not know if this is a medically correct description. It did contain one solid item, however: the little Ambien pill. "Well, I gave it a try," I thought. It seemed that any sleep I might get would have to come naturally.

I rang a second time for the nurse. Upon arriving, she emptied my pan and rinsed it clean. When she gave it back to me, I still felt rotten, so I arranged the pan and myself in the established anticipatory positioning. At this point, I believe I had entered into a state of delirium or some sort of condition of semi-consciousness. Anywise, I was not so far gone as to be unable to recognize the abrupt arrival of the next round of disgorging. I was surprised that the second episode was more voluminous and violent than the first. That was the bad news. The good news was that I earned great relief from the experience. After having to trouble a nurse for a second time to help with cleaning up, I did not even take back the pan after she had finished. I knew I would no longer need the pan's services. I was done. I had done everything Dr. Leonard had ordered. It was my hope that I had avoided vomiting long enough that the intended effect of the antibiotics was not compromised. The doc would tell me later that it was not. I soon fell asleep, and I slept surprisingly well, considering what awaited me on the following day. And a big day it would be, being it was likely to reveal much of what I could expect of the rest of my life.

CHAPTER SIX

Monday, Monday. So Good to Me?

I WAS AWAKENED ON Monday morning by what I came to regard to as my hospital alarm clock, of a rather ghastly sort. Starting on the previous morning, a member of the blood drawing crew showed up to draw blood from me every morning at between five and five-thirty, right through the last day of my stay. For a guy who is rather squeamish about needles, I sure had to put up with a lot of them. I was beginning to feel like a human pincushion.

Once awake on surgery day, there was no going back to sleep. Even though I had no breakfast to look forward to, I was eager to get the day going, not that I had any *real* power in pushing time and events forward to my satisfaction. Anyway, I was still hoping for a cancellation that would allow me to get into surgery during the morning. In addition to simply wanting the surgery behind me, I wanted the pathologists to get to work on the tumor so that I could know if it was benign or malignant. In spite of my pessimism, I still clung to the chance that the thing might turn out to be benign.

At around seven o'clock, one of my attending nurses informed me that my surgery would definitely *not* be before late morning, at the earliest. Having no reason to doubt the nurse's word, I immediately called Eva to let her know that she did not need to rush to the hospital. She, of course, wanted to know how I survived the nausea of the previous night. I gave her the high points of what transpired after she had gone home, assuring her that I was presently in good condition and ready for the surgery.

Eva was in my room just ahead of eight bells. When I eyeballed her, she seemed to be a tad nervous. That, of course, was to be expected. I, surprisingly, did not feel nervous. Fatalistic would be a better description of my state of mind that morning. And the truth be known, my attitude probably became describable as such soon after the word "tumor" became part of my lexicon of the moment.

Although we had discussed various legal considerations with our attorney friend on Easter Sunday afternoon, there were still a few things Eva and I needed to discuss before surgery. For instance, we agreed that I should not be kept on life support if things went wrong during the operation. I was not particularly worried about the surgery going fatally wrong, but there are no guarantees. As the consent form states, the practice of medicine and surgery are not exact sciences. The risk factor was driven home a few weeks after my surgery. A close friend and former colleague of mine underwent a heart related surgery that is considered routine, nowadays. Somehow, his lungs could not tolerate the procedure, and they failed. He died. Even though the odds are in the surgery patient's favor, someone has to be that one in ten thousand, or whatever the ratio might be. My friend was that one.

We also decided that if the surgeon saw something unexpectedly wrong once he started poking around my insides, our consent to attempting to fix it would be dependent upon the benefit being substantially greater than the risk. I believe that this thinking is commonly applied to surgery, generally.

The third and final scenario we considered was Eva's brainchild. She surprised me considerably when she asked, "What about if they say you should have a colostomy? Should I tell them to do it? Could you handle that?"

I thought for a short time. During this span of time, I thought about Brian Holst very recently telling a group of guys we breakfast with on Saturdays that his uncle has "the bag" and is one of the most fit and active guys he knows. I answered her question, "Yes. I could handle it."

Once satisfied that we had an idea of how to deal with the unforeseen or the unthinkable, Eva and I went into a holding pattern as we waited for my being called down to surgery. At around nine o'clock, Dr. Leonard stopped in for a quick visit to look me over one last time before surgery. I told him about my struggle to keep the antibiotics down and that I avoided vomiting until about eleven p.m. The doc did not seem concerned. Furthermore, he commented that my surgery would not occur before early afternoon, probably around one or one-thirty, with any luck. Like most folks past the age of six, I have learned to wait in lines for any number of reasons, like getting into the movies or checked out of the grocery store, for instance. But this would be the first time I had to wait in line to be operated on. "Why not?" I mentally commented. After all, I had already played host to a tumor and suffered from severe anemia for the first time. My intuition also insisted that I would be in for other "firsts," too.

The thing about waiting is that a person has time to think during the wait. In my case, I gave brief consideration to complications arising during my surgery due to my blood count. Dr. Leonard had told me that surgery is one thing with a blood count between ten and fifteen, but it is altogether a much riskier thing if the patient's blood count is under ten. Although my count was not much over ten, it was over this threshold. To my thinking, this meant that I would not likely die on the surgeon's table due to blood count related problems. Another point to ponder concerned the likelihood of my dying due to some complication mentioned on the consent form that I had signed. At this point, I had yet to personally know anyone who had died in surgery. Certainly this sort of thing happens, hence the mandatory consent form. The odds, though, were comfortably in my favor. Another possibility was that the surgeon, upon opening me up, would find that I was polluted with cancer, perhaps to some hopeless extent. Again, I did not personally know of anyone who fit this description, but I had heard of such cases. Even though I did not think this would be my case, I still had to acknowledge that it was possible.

I should make special mention of one particularly bizarre thought that ran through my mind as I awaited surgery: Nobody had the authority to make me go through with the operation, nobody at all. As an adult of legally sound mind, I had the option of simply getting up, getting dressed and getting a cab home. My imagined rebellion, of course, made no sense whatsoever. Counterproductive to the extreme, the thought was nothing more than the product of my deep frustration with my medical condition. Being an independent sort, I loathe being dictated to by anyone, and there I was being dictated to by a tumor, of all things! Fate can be so cruel. When reason returned, it forced me to acknowledge that my only sensible course of action was a surgery that would liberate me from the tyrant within me, a tyrant that would most assuredly kill me if left to wreak its havoc. Besides, Eva and I had a pact, of sorts. We had agreed that we would contend with this ordeal together and fight this battle "for us." I could never allow a snit to lead me into violating this pact and, thereby, heaping hurt and trauma on Eva. To do so would have been indefensible and unforgivable.

Having one's mortality shoved into one's face provides cause to contemplate the nature of life and its ultimate end. I was no exception. As I lay in my bed during the long wait, I had ample opportunity to consider the destinations to which my contemplative travels along the winding roads of philosophy and theology had led me. Essentially, I needed to satisfy myself that I was on firm footing in regards to these endeavors that seek to define the human condition. I was hoping that I did not feel compelled to rethink the philosophical and theological positions that I had developed over the years, especially the theological ones. Such rethinking would have been an admission that I believed the way that I had lived my life was wrong. This admission would have made me very insecure at facing the prospect of my life being soon over. No such admission was necessary. I wondered if I would feel the same way as I was being wheeled to surgery.

As is her modus operandi, Eva kept herself meaningfully busy during the wait. Besides always checking on my condition and needs, she kept certain people informed as to what was (or was not) going on. My mother, of course, was among that number of certain people. I know that my troubles were particularly hard on my mother because she felt additionally helpless due to her being so far away. Although it is true that she would have been just as helpless had she been in my room, my mother would have preferred to be close to the situation *just in case* being present might offer an opportunity for her to positively influence things. I talked with my mother briefly during Monday's marathon wait. She offered me encouragement by telling me that she had "a good feeling" about how all of this would turn out. She also advised me that I needed to be right with God going into this surgery. Mother was nervous. What could be more natural?

I watched one o'clock come and go.

I watched one-thirty come and go.

I grinned and recalled Dr. Leonard's judicious counsel that the surgery department runs on "its own time."

Around two o'clock, one of the shift nurses leaned into my room and announced that three o'clock was "show time." Three o'clock. Under normal circumstances, I would likely be getting home from work at about three, eager to get into my garage and begin my exercise set du jour. My goal would be to start exercising by the time Jeopardy started at three-thirty. Setting up a cable-fed television in the garage was Eva's idea, and a darn good one, too. In addition to exercising to Jeopardy and Seinfeld re-runs, I very much enjoyed exercising while a good sporting event was on, especially football. On this Monday, however, I was a contestant in a game that made me to wonder just how much jeopardy I was really in. Back in the fifties, one might have said, "*That's* the sixty-four thousand dollar question."

Just ahead of three o'clock, two women I had never seen entered my room. Their being strangers to me did not prevent my instant recognition that they were from surgery and that they came to take me there. They struck me as being very competent in performing such deliveries. In fact, on the heels of a quick statement of their purpose, they concluded that I would be best transported in the very bed in which I lay. I was literally rolling to surgery within two minutes of these ladies' arrival. Eva was following closely behind. It would not have been advisable to be in front of my bed as my chauffeurs pushed and pulled me along. To be sure, these gals meant business. I knew that I was headed to the authorized-personnel-only elevators because these were the elevators previously used to take me to my medical examinations conducted on the previous Friday. The staff of fourth floor west shot looks in my direction as I passed them. Most, if not all of them, knew where I was headed and the reason, too. I judged their looks as being sorrowfully sympathetic, but encouraging. I got the feeling they were rooting for me, but their professionalism and professional experience mandated they remain emotionally reserved. One nurse-to-be, a young lady named Robin, was on my right as I passed her. In one of those moments when two people can simultaneously read each other's mind, she and I extended our right hands toward one another and shook hands, thumbs-locked style. She was the last familiar person I remember seeing as I neared the elevators. At this point, my feeling was that of great trepidation. In fact, I felt this way from the moment the transport ladies showed up at my room, and I would continue to feel this way until the relaxation drug I would soon be given took effect. There was a lot of talking going on around me, but I said nothing. I found silence to be a source of strength, and I feared that if I spoke I would lose my strength. The only time I was tempted to speak was when there was something of a miniature fiasco regarding who had the right-of-way regarding the first available elevator: me or some woman with an empty cart that was about the size of a TV tray. I thought, "For heaven's sake woman, give it up, will ya'? Can't you see that I'm on my way to surgery, for crying out loud?" But I said nothing. My two attendants made the point for me, and the four of us were soon descending to the surgery department.

Once the elevator's doors opened, it was a short distance to surgery. The two women who delivered me seemed to have magically vanished as two nurses raced one another to take possession of me. They raced one another for me as if I were a fumbled football and they were opposing players. Although feigned to an extent, these two nurses were not completely unserious about getting to me first. By their own remarks, I came to know that they were lacking for work and desperate for something to do. This puzzled me because I had imagined surgery to have been very busy that day. I figured that, if anything, personnel in these parts would be displaying signs of wear and tear associated with a hectic day. One of the reasons I would have preferred my surgery be performed in the morning was that I calculated that folks would be fresh and on top of their games at the start of the business day. I was somewhat concerned about being on the tail end of the day's surgeries. But the two women now in a race to take custody of me seemed as fresh as morning dew. The nurse who looked like a former vice principal at my high school won the race and staked her claim of jurisdiction. I cannot recall her name. Defeated, but cooperative, the losing nurse helped the winning nurse wheel my bed into the preparation room. It was at this point in my journey that I could not believe my eyes. As my new bed drivers negotiated the turn around the corner of the counter that seemed to establish the border of the facility's command center, I made eye-to-eye contact with one of my recently abandoned chemistry students. Her name is Kristen. She is a good kid and a good student, but I truly did not care to encounter a student of mine who had just been read my farewell letter earlier that day. Again, I said nothing. I simply elevated my left hand by raising my forearm to be perpendicular to the bed's surface, and then I waved my four fingers four or five times in Kristen's direction. She made no noticeable response that I could discern. I think she was shocked. We were soon out of one another's sight as my bed came to rest in a room I thought was a bit undersized but, nonetheless, the prep room. Eva took a position at my upper left. Behind and above me was a window. I periodically tilted my head backward to get a glimpse of the out-of-doors. The weather was clear.

The two surgery prep nurses were real balls of fire. There was a lot of amiable chatter going on as they performed their duties, but I remained silent, except to answer their questions. I did not talk to Eva, either. If she would ask how I was doing, I would weakly answer "OK," or simply nod my head. The winning nurse, who was now doing most of my prep work, tried several times to get me to engage in her humor. Although I was not offended by it, I really was totally, completely and absolutely uninterested in humor. When she saw that in spite of her best efforts that I would not bite, she commented in a very sympathetic tone, "I know this is stressful." I appreciated her acknowledgement, and I remained silent.

Doc Leonard stopped in briefly. I assured him that I was "hanging in there," and he assured me that he would next see me in surgery.

Every now and again, I could see Kristen and some other high school aged kid working by stocking what appeared to be towels and linens in the proper storage bins that were built into the aforementioned counter. As Kristen passed my room in the course of performing her job, I think she tried to steal glimpses of me, perhaps to confirm that her eyes had not played a trick on her a few minutes prior. On the last pass I remember her making past my room, and just as she was leaving my range of sight, she called out, "Hi, Mr. Gaudio." I said nothing in reply. I had no wish to be rude. I just thought this teacher-student situation very awkward. Mere moments earlier, I had considered asking that the curtain be drawn along the window wall running parallel to the outside corridor so that Kristen could not see me. Then I thought that this was just one of the hazards of teaching in the community in which one lives. To be fair to Kristen, I am not particularly thrilled when I run into students or parents or colleagues at, for instance, some local restaurant, either. My undying preference is to keep my personal and professional lives separate, and I feel no guilt from it.

As expected, the anesthesiologist, a guy roughly my age, stopped by to interview me about things related to my being anesthetized. Upon entering my prep room, he introduced himself as "Rick," as opposed to Dr. Carstens. Since I would have expected Rick to introduce himself as doctor, I did not upon introduction appreciate that I was talking to my anesthesiologist. I thought he was another nurse who came to help in my being prepped for surgery. Rick surprised me a second time when he informed me that he would also have the additional responsibility of installing my epidural. This caught me off guard because I had assumed Dr. Leonard would set up the epidural. As it turned out, Dr. Leonard established what my pain management system would be, but he would only set up the pain-ball portion of it. Who installed what portion of my pain control system really did not matter to me, however, as long as the system worked effectively.

I had forgotten all that went into getting a patient prepped for the knife. Although longer than I expected, I did not suspect the time taken to prep me was unusually long because everything seemed to be going smoothly regarding my preparation. The only matter that probably took a little extra time was the changing of my IV needle. By this point in my prep, the two nurses who were initially in competition for me had become a team, and they were now making a coordinated effort to expedite my preparation. Upon closer inspection of my IV needle, they concluded that it was best switched for a larger one. Judging from their comments, it was better that I had a larger IV needle just in case a greater flow of some solution was desirable during surgery. It made sense to me that enough would be going on during surgery without having to hassle with something like changing an IV needle. The switch to a larger size was made easily, thankfully. I cannot recall if I ever saw the movie *The Panic in Needle Park*, but it is a safe bet I will not be renting it any time soon.

The last thing I remember during my prep is the nurse who began my prep saying it is time I get the "I don't care about anything drug." Maybe the larger IV needle allowed for such a large flow of this drug that I fell under its influence almost at the moment of its entry into my vein. I do not remember *anything* from the point of the above mentioned comment until I received a command from the surgery nurse sometime after I had been taken to the actual surgery room. The "I don't care...drug" *really* works. Take it from me. As further proof of its power, Eva told me that I had delivered a very serious lecture about the workings of the solar system to my captive audience. And she said it was very impressive. I regret having absolutely no recollection of my stellar performance. Also, I was surprised to learn that I had picked this subject upon which to lecture. Something to do with chemistry would have been logical. But I do not think that logic and this feel-good drug are necessarily compatible. I was just glad that I did not start to babble about something embarrassing, although I have to believe that the surgery prep folks have a policy something like, "What's said in surgery, stays in surgery."

Eva was so deeply stressed at this stage of things that she cannot recall our last words to one another as I approached the double doors of the surgery room. To be truthful, I suspect that I was in such a high orbit at this point that I might well have been incapable of any type of exchange of farewells. Farewells or not, the double doors meant that Eva and I had to part company. The next several hours would be much harder on Eva than on me.

It had to be soon after I entered the surgery room that a male nurse named Shawn directed me to sit at the edge of whatever I was on with my legs dangling. He assisted me in assuming this position, and then directed me to tilt my head downward, lean forward and rest the top of my head against his chest, assuring me that he would not allow me to fall. Shawn had accompanied Rick when he came to get my data for my anesthetic. Even under the influence of the no-worries drug, I recalled that Shawn looked like he could play middle linebacker in the NFL. Although I was about as limp as a rag doll, he would have no trouble preventing my falling off my perch. Months later, I realized that I had been repositioned so that my back was exposed, permitting Rick to install my epidural. I remember nothing of the epidural system being affixed to me. Once my head was positioned against Shawn's chest, I fell into a state of complete oblivion.

CHAPTER SEVEN

The Shakies

WHEN I REGAINED consciousness in the recovery room, I recall lying on my right side and shaking violently. It seemed as if I was lying on the surface of some sort of contraption designed to shake someone until his or her teeth rattled. Additionally, my mouth felt as if every molecule of water had vacated. In fact, the dryness was excessive to the extent that I had difficulty forming words. Nonetheless, I was able to call out, "I'm shaking." I must have assumed someone was present to hear me because I saw no one. The truth is I cannot even recall if my eyes were open at the time.

A woman's voice replied, "Do you have the chills or the shakies?"

I had never heard of the shakies, but I knew instantly that I had them, and not the chills. So, I answered, "The shakies."

Again, the same woman's voice: "Then it is the drugs. You're coming off the drugs. You'll be OK in a little while"

I must have been experiencing what a drug addict feels when going through detoxification. I would imagine that not even the mighty Shawn could have shaken me so violently for so long.

There was still the matter of my thirst. My throat was so dry that it seemed clogged or fused shut, making talking very difficult.

"My mouth is very dry. May I have some water?" I desperately asked.

"No. You can't have any water, right now. You're only allowed a few chips of ice," was the answer.

Again, the voice was that of the same woman, and I assume that it was she who inserted a chip or two of ice into my mouth. I am forced to make this assumption because I cannot recall ever seeing anybody in the recovery room.

After the much appreciated ice chips, the next thing I remember is being back in room 4006. My guardian angel was there, of course. Some lady connected to the recovery room was good enough to inform Eva of my imminent departure. This information allowed Eva to accompany me from recovery to my room. I would come to appreciate that it is not always easy for a concerned party to keep track of a surgery patient. Weeks after my surgery, a very good friend of ours found that trying to determine if his wife (also a very good friend) was in surgery or recovery to be an exercise in frustration.

Although never frustrated in her attempts to track me, Eva did have quite a scare thrown into her during the course of my surgery. As Eva relates it, the incident "scared the hell out of me (her)."

Still working to keep folks posted as to my status, Eva had abandoned the waiting room for the hallway. She thought the hall to be a more courteous and private venue for a telephone call to her mother. While getting my mother-in-law up to speed, she saw Dr. Leonard hurrying down the hallway in her direction. She immediately terminated the phone call and looked expectantly toward the doctor. Each was surprised to see the other, but Eva's surprise bordered fright as she wondered, "What's the doctor doing out here?"

Understanding that my wife was jolted by his presence, the doc stopped to explain it to her. As it was, Dr. Leonard was following my tumor and a length of my small intestine (about three inches) that he had ordered to pathology. He wanted to eyeball his work under a microscope. Even though such an examination could not provide him with a definitive answer regarding the completeness of the tumor's removal, his endeavor was still prudent. The urgency of the situation demanded the doctor not tarry, and he bolted to the lab. At least Eva now knew that the doc's presence outside the operating room was a matter of expediency as opposed to emergency.

Dr. Leonard, understandably, did not remain in the pathology lab for long. Consequently, he again encountered Eva on his return to surgery. This time, and without stopping, he informed Eva that he was both reasonably confident that he had gotten the whole tumor and that it was a stromal tumor. Stromal had no meaning to Eva (or me) at that time. Times would change.

Eva informed me that I got back to my room from surgery at about six thirty. I have absolutely no recollection of my arrival. The only definite recollections I have came well into the night, when I was alone in my darkened room. As I lay on my back with my legs slightly spread and my arms at my sides, I remember thinking that I was not in any pain. In fact, I felt comfortable. The pain management system must be working, I gratefully concluded. Furthermore, as my newly regained cognizance expanded, I became aware of something different about my nose, specifically my left nostril. At first I was perplexed, but then I remembered that Dr. Leonard had told me during a pre-surgery conversation that I would have a nasogastric (NG) tube as part of my anatomy upon leaving surgery. Truthfully, I did not really understand what such a device is. Moreover, I was only half listening to the doc as he enumerated the various details of my operation. I was simply too stunned by the fact that I was going to need to be operated on to pay much attention to the details of the event. My sense was that I was going to take a pounding and that I would deal with the aftermath of my surgery as necessary. Had I any prior experience with a NG tube, I doubtlessly would not have been so nonchalant about this medical device. Essentially, a NG tube is a flexible tube passed through a nostril (my left one) and down through the nasopharynx and esophagus, finally ending up in the stomach. Dr. Leonard intended that this tube would remove stuff from my stomach, probably mostly poisonous fluids. Its use can be the reverse of my situation, allowing for the input of nutrients into the stomach of a patient who cannot take food or drink by mouth.

In the days to come, I would begin to wonder which one was worse, the tumor or the NG tube. But at this point in my recovery, the tube was not yet bothersome to any notable extent.

Another of my first post surgery recollections was my sight being fixated on the top of an item of furniture positioned several feet away from the foot of my bed and toward my left. This piece of furniture was rather tall because it served as a combination of bureau, closet and shelving. For some reason, I found staring in this manner relaxing, even comforting. I have to conclude that the combination of various drugs that were permeating my body to different extents had much to do with my state of mind. In any event, I grew very empathetic in my trance like state. I *just knew* that once I got back on my feet again that I would have to do some sort of volunteer work at the hospital.

The last thing I remember pondering in the darkness was appreciating that I had been drawing strength form the well wishes and prayers of others as I endured my ordeal. Prior to my hospitalization, I would have had little, if any, expectation of there being power in the expressions of concern from others. Being a sports fan, I should have expected and understood this phenomenon. After all, a team typically plays its best in its home stadium or on its home court, in the presence of hordes of well wishing (some even praying) fans.

It seems that I considered these things for a long while, but I do not know for sure really how long before falling asleep. When I awoke to the morning's light, I took special note of the way it shone through block glass windows above the bathroom vanity and interacted with the earth tone colors of my room. I found the effect of this interplay of sunlight and color to be very soothing. Even though I had paid no attention to this light and color show prior to surgery, I came to look forward to it each of the remaining mornings of my hospitalization, which would turn out to be six. For many years it has been my habit to begin days as tranquilly as possible. Doing so helps me to feel under control and better able to face whatever the day might deliver.

Tuesday would deliver the need for me to get out of bed for the first time after surgery. I was concerned, to say the least, about the degree of pain I would have to endure in the early stages of my convalescence. As I lay practically motionless in bed, I felt quite comfortable. Pain was not a problem. Getting up and moving around, though, promised to be "a whole 'nother ball game." To be honest, I was not looking forward to the physical therapist's scheduled arrival at around nine o'clock. I found the thought of getting out of bed to be a bit scary. But the thought of clotting blood frightened me even more.

Eva arrived early Tuesday morning, eager to see how I weathered the night. It was as hard for her to see me in such a battered state as it was for me to accept it. She fussed over me, doing anything she could think of doing to try to make me more comfortable, like arranging my pillows more to my liking. I was still on an ice-chips-only diet, and she was always at the ready to meet my every request for another serving. Strangely, I had lost my craving for food because I had no sense of hunger. This would be the case for about the next forty-eight hours. But when my appetite returned, it would do so in spades.

Unlike my appetite, my thinking had retuned to normal. I was cognizant of all that was going on around me, and I was fully coherent. This is not to suggest that I consider my thinking of the previous night to have been incoherent, only that it had the property of exceptional serenity.

The physical therapist showed up as scheduled. Her name was Laura, and she had an assistant named James. He was in some stage of training to be a nurse. One of my floor nurses also arrived with Laura and James. These folks were all present to help me to take the longest short walk of my life.

Laura was talkative and rather expressive. She was task oriented, too. After a quick introduction and "How-do-you-do?" Laura had me engaged in doing stretching exercises for my feet and legs as she peppered me with questions about what I felt and where I felt it. The stretching was to help prepare me for my first post surgery steps. While giving me instruction in the correct method of doing my stretching, Laura pulled away the bed covers. Since the gown I was wearing only covered my legs to my knees, my legs were now visible from the knees down. Taking note of the size of my calve muscles, Laura unabashedly complimented me and predicted that these muscles would expedite my return to bipedal locomotion. Although I smiled at her compliment, I was inwardly sad that it would be eight to ten weeks before I could expect to be allowed to put my legs through the paces to which they had become accustomed.

The main difficulty in getting me out of bed was not yours truly, I am happy to be able to say. The truth is that the biggest problem in getting me onto the floor was figuring out how to accommodate the collection of equipment to which I was connected. Fortunately, James came to the rescue.

James had been a commercial pilot but decided he wanted a career change. As one might expect of a pilot, James had an ability to quickly evaluate a problem and solve it. In my case, the problem was the aforementioned gaggle of equipment to which I was connected via various tubes and wires. Specifically, this collection of stuff had to become my shadow, of sorts, when I traveled. Complicating the matter, the equipment was distributed on two separate rolling IV trees located on either side of the head of my bed. Getting me out of bed while I was connected to all this stuff (IV solutions, blood oxygen monitor, epidural apparatus, morphine dispenser, NG tube pump, catheter) was a little like Lemuel Gulliver (in *Gulliver's Travels*) trying to free himself from the web of tie-downs that the Lilliputians used to constrain him.

No need to fear. James took stock of the situation and straight away went to work on a solution. We four observers (including Eva) were amazed at the rapidity with which James consolidated all of my medical tagalongs onto a single IV tree. Furthermore, this consolidation was a model of organization, in that all things were placed in a logical and secure position on the tree. I would benefit from James' organizational genius for days to come.

After all of us sincerely expressed our appreciation for James' efforts, I started in earnest to depart my bed. Receiving assistance in some form or another from the three medical persons present, I eventually found myself extricated. To be sure, I was a bit shaky and needed a walker for support, but I was on my feet. It took the better part of ten minutes to get me upright, but speed was not the objective of this game. And besides, the medical equipment (not I) consumed most of the ten minutes.

Along the way to getting me in a standing position, I was continually asked about the extent to which I was experiencing pain. When asked, I was to report my pain as being along a scale from zero to ten, ten representing the greatest severity. To be truthful, I must say that my pain was not too tough. I never called out a number higher than two and a half. The worst pain occurred as I moved my feet from my bed to the floor, and vice versa. All told, my feeling of frailty exceeded my feeling of pain. I was growing increasingly appreciative of the pain management system Dr. Leonard had devised for me.

"Wow," was my first thought once I finally assumed a standing position. I was deeply stunned. Merely getting me out of bed had required the considerable energy and expertise of a small group of people. Furthermore, the formerly automatic act of standing now necessitated that I use a walker for support. Not too many days prior, and even in an anemic state, I could easily kick a forty-pound heavy bag with no modest amount of force. I felt like a shell of my former self. Even after the hemorrhoidectomy I had almost twenty-one years earlier, walking was no problem, although that surgery was not without its own unique post surgery pain.

It should be noted that what I am referring to here as "standing" is not to convey an image of perfectly straight posture. In fact, I was bent over like an old man.

Laura was no rookie to the physical therapy business, so she did not press me excessively. She only wanted my best effort under the circumstances as she urged me to stand as straight as possible. I think that had I jerked my torso perfectly perpendicular to the floor, I would have taxed the pain ball and epidural to a point that I would have regretted. The first walking I did after getting home from the hospital I did over a course I designed in my backyard. Eva would spy on me while I would dutifully do my back yard walking. Weeks after I had returned to walking normally, Eva told me that I walked in a noticeably stooped fashion for several weeks after getting home.

My first walk was to be of a distance that I felt manageable. Taking my initial walker assisted steps, I had no idea what this distance would measure, exactly, but I knew that its measure would be short. As it turned out, I walked in a westward direction toward my room's door, maintaining a death grip on the handles of the walker, which had become, in my view, a barrier between my belly and the rest of the world. I made it to the door, a distance of about fifteen feet. Laura principally assisted me, and James, of course, steered the loaded-to-capacity IV tree that needed to make the trek, too. Once I actually got moving, I guess that it required me about thirty seconds to travel the fifteen feet. Recognizing that this was not a one-way trip, I figured that I had gone far enough from my bed for my first outing. After making my decision known to all present, I began to turn myself around for the return trip. Even though this first expedition did not constitute much of a hike, it was an important step toward my goal of a complete recovery.

Getting back into bed would turn out to be the most painful part of this exercise session, and subsequent ones, too. Although it was painful to accomplish, at least gravity was in my favor when I was getting out of bed. On the way back into it, I would have to fight gravity, which added to my difficulty. Most of this fight took the form of lifting my legs into the bed. In performing this maneuver, I was gaining a first hand appreciation for an observation that Dr. Leonard would make in the coming days. It was something to the effect that "Blinking is about the only thing you do that doesn't require the use of your stomach muscles." Think about it.

Once I had safely returned to my bed, Laura offered her observations and opinions regarding my brief stroll. Although generous with her praise for my efforts, Laura emphasized that I was not to rest on my laurels. She prescribed that I get out of bed routinely each day and try to accomplish a longer, stronger walking session each time.

I understood, and I agreed to be diligent in doing my assignments, like any good student would. We exchanged farewells, and Laura left. James and the floor nurse had left earlier, in fact soon after I had gotten back into bed. I would not see Laura again. Over the next five days, I worked with three different physical therapists, two young women and one young man. They were all very helpful in my recovery, especially a young lady named Monika.

The frailty to which I alluded above stemmed from the presence of the long incision running up my abdomen. Although I had not yet seen the actual cut, the length of the bandage allowed me to deduce that it ran vertically from an inch or so above my penis to about three inches above my belly button. The sight intimidated me. I was petrified by the thought of bumping it even slightly. Had it been possible, I would have had a baseball catcher's mask, or something very nearly resembling one, secured over my incision. My near paranoia about this gash along my gut would leave me jumpy for weeks to come. Until nearly the end of May, if anyone made any kind of motion I feared was headed toward my stomach area, I would flinch. I really do not think that I had ever felt so vulnerable. I imagined that I felt like a very old person would feel when venturing out into some fast paced, rough and tumble public venue, like a teachers' parking lot after school on a Friday. Specifically, I felt that my physical prowess had been reduced to nothing. Humbling, very humbling.

Through all of this business of my first post surgery exit from bed, the thing that I found to be most annoying had nothing to do with my medical condition. Instead, it had to do with my teaching specialty, i.e. chemistry. When I am asked what I do for a living, and I answer that I teach chemistry, I am sure to get some sort of response.

Sometimes, the questioner will express revulsion at the mere mention of chemistry. At other times, a person will actually want to talk some chemistry, especially if he or she has a fond memory stemming from having taken a high school or college chemistry course. In the case of the former type of person, I try to offer some consolation to soothe the harm done to the individual's psyche. In the case to the latter, I politely listen and, possibly, engage in a little chemistry chitchat.

Another category of person I inevitably encounter wants to impress me with his or her memorization of the periodic table or, more likely, some portion of it. I find this category of person to be annoying, to put it mildly. A woman who intruded upon my first post-surgery stroll tested my manners when she replied with gibberish when I answered her query, "What kind of work do you do?" Nobody present, in fact, had any idea what she had said as a response to my telling her that I teach chemistry. She seemed surprised that nobody could make sense of her gibberish, but she seemed down right disappointed in my case. She repeated, and mostly to me, her nonsensical statement a second time, and did so in a manner that a person would employ to coax an answer he or she knows is imbedded in another's memory. It was as if she were a mother drilling her fourth grade son on the states' capitals, knowing that he had on the day before correctly answered for a state, but currently could not retrieve the correct capital from his memory. Alas, I again failed to recognize the meaning of her sounds, finding no word among them that I could recognize. When the intruder perceived the situation as being hopeless, and I think viewing me as being somewhat pathetic, she revealed she had been vocalizing a mnemonic device she learned back in high school, which enabled her to remember the first twenty or so elements on the periodic table.

Big deal.

Memorization of the periodic table represents no measure of a person's chemical intelligence or elemental prowess, *whatsoever.* I, too, used to waste energy memorizing the table, and I mean *all* the elements and their symbols. I would do the same thing with the Pittsburgh Steelers' roster, i.e., memorize each player on the whole squad by his jersey number. One exercise was as useless as the other, except to maybe win a bar bet on occasion. Besides, if one is to memorize the periodic table, why stop with just the names and symbols of the elements? Why not memorize the elements' densities, melting and boiling temperatures, common oxidation states and the like? Memorizing the table requires no understanding of its connection to the cosmos, i.e., its depiction of physical reality. The act of merely memorizing the table is akin to a child's reading a legal document, perfectly pronouncing each word therein, but in fact understanding nothing of the document's meaning. The great Albert Einstein was unable to recall the speed of sound during a particular discourse. Some of those present were shocked at his lapse. Einstein simply shrugged it all off, puzzled as to why one would bother memorizing that which could be easily referenced. Referencing, by the way, would require considering the physical state of the medium, along with other factors. In other words, there is no single answer to the question, "What's the speed of sound?"

Another of my memories specific to Tuesday was that it was the day on which I came closest to losing my temper during my hospitalization. The cause of my angst was the NG tube, at least in an indirect sort of way. At this point, the tube was not as painful a presence as it would soon become. The trouble it presented at this juncture was more a matter of mechanics than one of pain. Specifically, each time I left the bed necessitated the tube be disconnected from its pump, which was located on the floor at the head of my bed and to my left as I lay. The system was designed such that a connecting joint in the tubing was located at a point along the tubing's length corresponding to my left rib cage about six inches northeast from my belly button. Twice on Tuesday, separating the two sections of tubing at this joint resulted in spillage from the tubing onto the part of my gown covering my left rib cage area. On each occasion, what spilled was a substantial volume of brownish liquid that had been pumped from my stomach. Yummy. Some of this stuff always remained in the tube, and it was plainly visible because the tubing was transparent. Thus confined, its presence was tolerable. But when allowed to escape its incarceration, its unsanitary presence was nothing short of obnoxious. Furthermore, spilled stomach fluid in the immediate vicinity of my incision was a situation ripe for infection. And I had enough trouble as things were, without the complication of dealing with an infection. After the second occurrence of spillage, it was obvious that an adjustment in technique was required to deal with the matter of disconnecting the joint in a more sanitary way. So, I made it my policy that before permitting anyone to disconnect me from the NG tube pump, a large towel, folded to a quarter of its total area, had to be placed under the joint. The folded towel, properly positioned, would shield me from any spillage, which, by the way, occurred on nearly each instance of disconnecting the joint. One of my attending nurses remarked that the problem that I was experiencing was not uncommon. This led me to wonder why some sanitation system similar to mine had not become standard practice before I had arrived on the scene. The problem was solved, but the NG tube was not finished making my life miserable just yet.

The goal of getting me up and walking was to reduce the chance of my suffering from blood clots. Another concern related to my recovery was keeping my lungs clear. To keep my lungs healthy, I would frequently use a device called a spirometer on each of the first six days following surgery. A spirometer is an odd-looking thing. Essentially, its component parts are a plastic housing, a piston and an attached length of flexible tubing. The free end of the tubing has a mouthpiece. Making the piston rise in its cylinder is done counter-intuitively, i.e., by *inhaling* through the tube. I soon made a game of this device's usage. My objective in the game was to force the piston to the maximum height allowed by the cylinder, and to achieve this at least once during a session of using the device. A session of usage consisted of five to ten separate attempts to force the piston to the ceiling of the cylinder. All I had to do in order to win a session was pin the piston against the cylinder's ceiling just once. And there were sessions in which I pinned the piston two or three times. All told, I probably won about two thirds of the sessions. There were, alas, times when no matter how hard I tried, I could not coax the piston up to the cylinder's ceiling even once. Nevertheless, I won even when I lost. This statement is defensible because even in defeat, my lungs were still getting the workout intended. And believe me when I say that an honest session of using one of these devices truly works the lungs. I did bring this device home with me, but I never used it outside the hospital, figuring my return to a normal life provided sufficient activity for my lungs.

I felt proud of my efforts on the first day following surgery. My recovery was going to be a rather lengthy journey, and my first steps, both literal and figurative, were an unqualified success in my view. Eva was pleased, too. I think that she was especially impressed with my attitude. Over the coming days and weeks, she would keep close tabs on both my physical and psychological states. I would do the same because I was more than eager to return to being my old self, warts and all, as soon as possible. Well, maybe with just a few fewer warts.

All three of my doctors visited me on Tuesday. The first up was Dr. Freudenburg. He stopped in well ahead of six that morning. With the exception of just two days on which he was unable to visit, Dr. Freudenburg came by each morning before six o'clock. I greatly appreciated his genuine concern for me. Dr. Freudenburg is a very nice man who happened to choose the profession of medical doctor. It is my opinion that it is his patients' good fortune that he made that choice. I am certain that he would have been very successful had he chosen to be an accountant, for example. In such an occupation, however, the world would have had a very much-reduced opportunity to benefit from the goodness of Dr. Freudenburg's heart.

Dr. Leonard stopped by later that morning. My first words to him were, "You sure hit hard, Doc." He laughed.

The doc gave me a rundown of what he did. I could tell that he viewed the surgery as having gone very smoothly, and he was pleased to say, and I to hear, that he had every reason to believe that the tumor had been entirely removed. He described the tumor's size as being "golf ball plus." In doing some research later, I learned that the type of tumor I had could grow to be very much larger than a golf ball. Furthermore, Doc informed me that he gave my inner regions in the vicinity of the small intestine a thorough looking over. I was delighted to hear that he found no indication of cancer anywhere else that it might have figured to spread. It appeared that my uninvited boarder had been restricted to one small room, so to speak, prior to its eviction.

Next, the surgeon noted that the matter was now in the hands of pathology. His position was to let the pathology department take the time they deemed necessary to properly do their work. He wisely counseled, "We want an accurate report (from pathology), not a quick report." Looking in the doc's direction, I nodded in agreement. Although just a guess on my part, I mentally tagged Thursday as the earliest that I would definitively know whether the tumor was benign or malignant. As mentioned before, I decided to brace myself for a lab report of an undesirable kind. Nonetheless, I still wanted to definitively *know* one way or the other, good news or bad, and if bad, how bad.

All this time, the doc had been standing at the foot of my bed as we conversed. When he started to move to his left and motioned to me to remove my bed covers, I knew he wanted to look at my incision even before he said, "Let's have a look." I was not yet ready to see what I would have to live with for the rest of my life. So, instead of casting my eyes on the incision as Dr. Leonard pulled away the gauze bandage covering it, I looked steadily at the doc's face. I figured that I would be able to deduce the condition of my cut by the look it induced on the surgeon's face. The facial expression I observed would be best described as impassive. I interpreted this as a good sign. Dr. Leonard *expected* to see no problems with the incision. A look of surprise, and certainly one of shock, on the other hand, would have been cause for concern. After replacing the gauze, he examined the pain ball and was satisfied with it, too.

Before heading to perform his next duty, the doc prescribed that I should be active, but reasonably so. He conveyed that "slow and steady will win the race." I had to chuckle at the doc's choice of words because the image of my attempting any kind of footrace struck me as being humorously preposterous. This is not to suggest that I regarded Dr. Leonard's advice lightly, for I most certainly did not. In fact, I understood his point perfectly and intended to heed it.

In his typical who-was-that-masked-man fashion, the doc bolted when his business with me was completed. I knew without the doc's saying, however, that he intended to monitor me on a daily basis until he released me from the hospital.

Dr. Coff arrived in my room later that morning. I would classify his visit as being more social than medical in nature, more of a courtesy visit. His job was, after all, done. He had identified my problem and placed me in the hands of someone who was capable of solving it. The doc sincerely inquired as to how I was feeling, and he expressed optimism about my recovery, short term and long. Within a couple of minutes, he was bidding Eva and me farewell and went on his way. I would not see Dr. Coff again for the duration of my stay at LUH.

The combination of physical therapy, doctors' visits and frequent tending by nurses eventually wore me down, so I dozed for a while. By early afternoon, I was again awake. In my estimation, it was time to try a second round of walking. With assistance from Eva and a floor nurse, I was soon standing. Thanks to James' earlier work, getting out of bed this time was much faster. Relying heavily on my walker,

I headed toward the door. Boldly, I passed over its threshold, placing myself in the open space beyond. I felt a little weird being among all those bustling, able-bodied people, but this was as good a time as any to make my reentry into society, albeit on a small scale and in a very protected venue. I felt a bit like a celebrity as various medical folks I encountered offered me acknowledgement and encouragement. Eva was a little concerned that I would try to do too much, but I assured her that my hike would be a short one, and it was. A fair estimate of the length of my second stroll would be about one hundred feet, round trip. This distance would have been an insult to my legs under normal circumstances, but my circumstances were anything but normal. I had just traveled about four times the distance of my first exercise session, and I was content with my improvement. Progress was being made!

Instead of returning to my bed at trip's end, I decided to take a seat in one of the chairs in my room. Lying in bed all the time is rougher than it looks. Additionally, Eva told me that various problems could result from being bed bound for too long. For instance, a friend of ours who had been recently hospitalized developed a problem in the form of soreness in the heels of her feet due to being bedridden. How a problem with one's feet can arise from being in bed for too long is beyond me, but I was determined to avoid developing any problems with my feet or legs. I would tolerate nothing getting in the way of my walking exercises, no matter how feeble my steps. I viewed walking not only as the main means by which to restore my physical health, but it was also going to play a key role in helping me to preserve my sanity.

If asked to describe through Tuesday how I felt, psychologically speaking, I would have to reply that it seemed a bit like I was in an episode of The Twilight Zone. Plots of this TV classic often involved characters feeling stunned and at a loss to explain things. I sure was stunned, and my tumor was not of the type easily explained. Furthermore, abnormality was the norm on The Twilight Zone. In my case, while in the hospital I had a very abnormal dream. I call it my "This is no dream, dream." Sometimes while experiencing an unpleasant dream, I am able to acknowledge that I am only dreaming and that I can escape the dream's unpleasantness by simply awakening. In the hospital, something occurred that was quite the opposite. Specifically, I dreamed that all of this hospital stuff I was enduring was real, and there would be no escape by awakening. I had never had such a dream previously. For instance, as a child, I had never been in trouble with my parents and dreamed that this trouble was no dream and that I would, in fact, have to deal with my folks when I awoke. Presently, when I look at the fresh scar running up my belly I often think or say aloud to myself, "This is no dream, Jimmy boy, no dream at all."

No more than twice on Tuesday, I self-medicated using the morphine machine, as I will call it. Again, during the entirety of my ordeal, I was never in anything approaching excruciating pain that was the direct result of my surgery. When I administered the morphine, it was only to see if its usage would push my pain (or discomfort) all the way down to zero. It did not. Frankly, I cannot say that I "felt" the morphine at all. Consequently, I may have tried it two or three more times through Thursday, before abandoning its usage completely. It is not my intention to imply that this morphine system is useless for all people all of the time. It may well be a godsend to some folks struggling with severe pain. I should also mention that the morphine machine of the type I had was designed to allow the administration of morphine at a prescribed rate, *only*. The dispensation system, in other words, was designed to prevent me (or any patient) from overdosing.

Wednesday and Thursday had much the same look as Tuesday. There were some differences, however.

One difference was that I was able to walk much better on Wednesday, and I improved in this exercise even more on Thursday. In fact, by Friday the walker would be of more interest to me in regards to its shielding benefit than its service as a prop.

Another difference that was specific to Thursday was that I went into the day expecting it would be the day of reckoning in regard to the pathology report. I was mildly disappointed, therefore, when neither Dr. Freudenburg, in the early morning, nor Dr. Leonard, later in the day, delivered news of the report. "Friday would be the day," I mentally guessed.

A third difference was the extent to which the NG tube was making its presence felt, and I mean the word "felt" as it relates to pain. My left nostril was becoming noticeably sorer, to be sure. My throat, however, was starting to kill me. By Thursday, I absolutely dreaded swallowing because my throat had become so terribly irritated. How would I have ever guessed that my *throat* would be the source of my worst pain following surgery on my *guts*? At this time, Dr. Leonard still only permitted me to ingest ice chips or lemon drops. His edict disallowed any consideration of my taking sore throat medication. Of course, neither ice chips nor lemon drops provided me with any real relief, and likewise for the morphine. In my condition, talking became too painful to justify, as far as casual conversation was concerned. So, I apologetically informed Eva that until the tube was removed, future conversations would have to be mostly one-sided. The maddening part of getting rid of the tube was that I could command that it be removed, provided that I could first perform *one specific act*.

Eva was very sympathetic to my misery, and she was determined to try to soothe it in some way or another. Ideally, she would have liked to eliminate the soreness in my throat in some fast acting, magical way. Since magic was not a viable option, she would try something more practicable: Diversion. Her intention was to offer to read the local newspaper to me. I did not know how well this would help to minimize my discomfort, but I did think that having Eva read aloud would help to remove some of the awkwardness caused by my being forced into a state of muteness. The readings would begin with Eva offering headlines of articles until I indicated that one interested me. She would then read the article in its entirety, unless I lost interest. Sometimes I would lie in bed as she read, and sometimes I would be seated in a chair. In order to concentrate on the article's content, I would lock my sight onto some fixed point in the room or watch Eva's face as she read. To my surprise, these reading sessions helped me to cope with my throat. Just being silent was helpful, of course, and focusing on following the flow of the article as Eva read it significantly diverted my attention from my throat, as intended. I again found myself in Eva's debt, but we both knew that the true solution to the torture I was enduring lay in the tube's removal.

So, Thursday brought me no news of pathology's findings nor did it bring me relief from the NG tube. I expected better of the morrow.

CHAPTER EIGHT

Friday the 13th

PAR FOR THE course, I got little sleep Thursday night. I would have especially appreciated a good night's sleep as a means by which to escape my nagging sore throat for a time. But the typical hospital activity through the night would only permit me a session of sleep describable as fitful. Ironically, I was, in fact, asleep when John, a tall, lanky member of the blood drawing crew, awakened me at about five-thirty Friday morning to draw his department's daily due. Even though annoyed at being awakened after so little sleep, I still attempted to be politely tolerant of John's need to do his job. I explained that I had a very sore throat, and asked John to excuse my reluctance to engage in small talk. As I lay with my left arm surrendered to John, I was more asleep than awake when Dr. Freudenburg walked into the room.

"Hey, Doc," I managed, as he neared the foot of my bed, following with "What's up?"

"You got some very good news this morning," was his reply to my query.

"Oh? Please tell me more," I requested, sleep and throat soreness no longer of import to me.

He did.

"Your pathology report is good," the doc started, then concluded with, "Once you get out of here, you'll probably go on living the next twenty-five years of your life like nothing happened, except for needing to recover from the surgery."

I wanted to call Eva, then and there. It's amazing how a dose of good news can chase one's ills.

"This *is* good news," I concurred, but in the moment of my little miracle, I did not think to ask the doc if his optimism was based on the tumor having been classified as benign in the pathology report.

As usual, the doc did not stay long. Obviously pleased to have served in the role of the messenger bearing good news, Dr. Freudenburg bid me farewell and took his leave, coffee mug in hand.

Eva arrived just ahead of eight o'clock. I wasted no time in relaying the good news. My words caused her whole face to light up, and she eagerly pressed me for details, more than I could provide. My wife can rapid-fire questions like a machine gun. None of her queries, though, sought to establish the tumor's classification as benign.

On a Friday so dreaded by the superstitious, Eva and I were feeling blessed with good luck. Such a wonderful turn of events had me thinking that I could leave the hospital, once discharged, concerning myself with recovering from the surgery and nothing more. It seemed that I had once again dodged a bullet on the battlefield of life.

Dr. Leonard was in pretty early that morning, and I am sure it was because he wanted to get the news of the pathology report to me, sooner than later. When he entered the room, he found Eva and me in high spirits. Although my throat was still plenty sore, it was not able to negate the good feeling in my soul. The infusion of adrenalin provided by Dr. Freudenburg's visit was having a similar effect on my state of alertness.

The doc took hold of the back of a chair and positioned it to his liking near the foot of my bed. Soon after seating himself, he proclaimed, "Well, you have reason to be very happy today."

"So I hear, Doc," I responded, following with the explanation, "Dr. Freudenburg told me about the pathology report earlier this morning."

Doc nodded, then offered his interpretation of my medical odyessy, as he saw it, at least to date. In his view, when the tumor was first discovered I was in the "Uh-oh" stage. Once he opened me up, he described me as having improved to the "This isn't as bad as it could have been" stage. With the delivery of the pathology report, he placed me in the "You've got a lot to be thankful for" stage.

For a reason I cannot explain, the "second stage" of my journey, as viewed by the doc, struck a chord with me. There was something about the way Doc said these words that made me understand how close to the precipice I had veered. I could have been in a state of free fall, approaching terminal velocity, instead of basking in the good news of the day. Sobering. Very sobering.

Continuing our discussion, Dr. Leonard described my tumor using terms like "self-contained" and "highly organized." My medical expertise is limited, to be sure, but I liked those descriptions. I surmised that had the tumor been of the opposite descriptions, this Friday falling on the thirteenth day of April would have had a much less festive feel to it. The description of benign, though, was still lacking.

Dr. Leonard went on to inform me that he was going to refer me to an oncologist, a Dr. Barnett, in fact. The mention of an oncologist took me, and I am sure Eva, by surprise. The doc gave the impression that this referral was a precautionary measure, an attempt to cover all the bases. It seemed that the doc was saying that his specialty is *removing* tumors, not analyzing them or dealing with them as might be post-operatively necessary. As I understood things, I would meet this Dr. Barnett, whom Dr. Leonard described as not only being "one of the young bright ones," but also "very nice" (a rare combination, in the doc's words), and consult with him on an infrequent basis. Maybe this Dr. Barnett would be the guy keeping an eye on my innards over the next couple of years, or however long it would be prudent to monitor me.

I felt a little disappointed in learning that there needed to be another doctor in my future, an oncologist, nonetheless. Anyway, I could still feel good about what my doctors had told me this morning. It seemed that I had not only passed the tumor test, but I had earned a high score in so doing. The fact remained, nonetheless, neither doctor had referred to my tumor as being benign.

After another quick look at the handiwork the doc had left along my abdomen, he was waving and saying his farewells as he strode toward the world beyond my door. I was feeling very fortunate that fate had placed me in the hands of Dr. Leonard, surgeon most extraordinary.

"Well, was the tumor benign?" Eva asked me, on the heels of the doc's exit.

"Well why didn't you ask the doc when he was here?" I volleyed.

The answer to my question was simple, perhaps. The reason Eva had not asked the doctor was the same one for which *I* had failed to ask *either* doctor: The news sounded so good that we felt it implied that the tumor was benign. Perhaps , however, we were subconsciously afraid to ask

The remainder of Friday morning and all of the afternoon were occupied with the same routine of activities of the previous couple of days. The performance of my walking exercises could now legitimately be described as occurring frequently, and I was getting stronger with each session. On Friday, I was capable of walking up and down sets of practice steps located in the physical therapy room on my floor. Steps had returned to my daily life. The very constructions that had abruptly exposed my physical deterioration were now to expedite my return to normalcy. The irony was not lost on me. Like Gomer used to ask Andy, "Ain't life funny, Andy? Ain't life funny?" Shazam!

Despite my physical improvement and a favorable pathology report, I was developing a deepening hatred for the tube, and it was getting more difficult to distract myself from its presence, regardless of the activity in which I tried to immerse myself. To complicate matters, on Friday my appetite began to return. This made the NG tube's intrusion all the more frustrating because I could not eat anything other than ice chips and lemon drops until the tube was removed, Dr. Leonard's orders. I was beginning to loathe the tube.

Just when I thought I was about to scream or cry or jump out a window because of the increasing weight of my frustration, Dr. J. Mark Barnett stopped in for his first consultation. And it was near five o'clock on a Friday afternoon! I was impressed. It seemed that Dr. Barnett took his job seriously.

I figure Dr. Barnett to be somewhere between his middle and late thirties. He is tall, slender and handsome. His manner is properly described as congenial. He is instantly likable, as Dr. Leonard had said, and I was betting that the young doc was as talented as touted, too.

Doc politely introduced himself, as he got comfortable in a chair to my right. I was lying in bed at the time. I mentioned that Dr. Leonard had told me to expect a visit from an oncologist. In addition, I could not resist telling Dr. Barnett how it was his older colleague had described him. Dr. Barnett concurred when I remarked that such an opinion is a feather in his cap, since Dr. Leonard is not one to pass out accolades lightly. It was clear that Dr. Barnett is a modest man.

"So, it looks like you've been rather busy recently," was the way the doc characterized my life, medically speaking, over the last eight days.

"Yeah, and I can't believe I could have been so wrong about what was going on with me," I admitted.

I piqued the doc's interest with my vague confession enough that he asked, "How do you mean?"

"Well," I began, "I thought my problem had to do with somehow falling out of aerobic condition or developing some sort of bug." I finished cleansing my conscience with, "So I started to push myself harder in exercise as a solution. Turns out my prescription was about a hundred and eighty degrees wrong."

With a look and a tone that indicated Dr. Barnett thought that I was being too hard on myself, he asked rhetorically, "But how could you have been expected to suspect a well-hidden tumor was your problem?"

Those were just the right words spoken in just the right way. I felt less a fool. A psychiatrist could not have done a better job.

Purposefully taking my medical record or chart in his right hand, the doc began a formal recount of my recent medical history, in a point-by-point fashion. At times, it was almost as if the doc were asking me if I agreed with the way my record read. I am sure his method was designed to get himself up to speed and to gauge how his patient, whether that would be me or someone else, felt about the official accounting of events. "A smart approach," I thought, and one that I might well have used had I been in his shoes.

The thrust of Doc's visit was to inform me that other than keeping an eye on some of my internal organs' conditions in the future, my treatment had essentially been completed, in the form of what appeared to be a very successful surgery. Pursuant to making future examinations meaningful, he informed me that he would have me undergo another CAT-scan on Monday, in order to establish a baseline for my lungs to go along with the baselines established for my other organs of interest from prior scanning.

The doctor sincerely asked if Eva or I had any questions. Of course we did have one in particular. So one of us, I cannot remember who, asked the doc if the tumor was benign.

"No it wasn't," answered Dr. Barnett.

Hmmm.

The doc could see that we were at a loss for words, so he offered an explanation.

"Your tumor was technically malignant," he instructed, continuing with, "This means that it was cancerous and *could* have spread." Although my tumor was of the type that could have spread, it had *not*. This fact alone would have served as reason to rejoice. Additionally, it had not burst, neither before nor during surgery, either scenario being very undesirable.

"So," I thought, "these would be two good reasons Drs. Freudenburg and Leonard would be so pleased with my situation." There were other reasons, too.

Being medical doctors, Dr. Freudenburg and Dr. Leonard knew how to interpret a pathology report. This report, which I would finally see for myself in about a week, described my tumor as a gastrointestinal stromal tumor (GIST) of low malignant potential. The malignant potentials of GIST's are as follows: extremely low, low, moderate and high. These potentials are made considering the following facts or data: tumor size, cleanness of surgical margins, mitotic count.

The fact that my tumor had not spread, in conjunction with its size being a "large small" or a "small medium" and its showing clean (negative) surgical margins and its showing a mitotic count of five or less (four in my case), rendered it to be of low malignant potential.

The doctors had been justified in framing the particulars of my tumor as good news. Sure I would have preferred that the tumor was benign, but if it had to be cancerous, it looked like I had an easy version of malignancy. Although I had not dodged the bullet, it only seemed to have grazed me, stunning me without killing me.

Well, that was that. Now done with business, Dr. Barnett excused himself in as polite a way as he had introduced himself. He also informed me that a colleague of his would be in on Sunday to see me. The doc himself would again visit me on Monday, preferably after the scan that he would schedule for me on that morning.

Dr. Barnett and his wife were going out with Dr. Freudenburg and his wife for dinner that evening. I sincerely wished the dinner party a good time, and I asked Dr. Barnett to give my regards to Dr. Freudenburg. He consented and was on his way.

Eva and I were left to reevaluate our view of where I had been, where I currently was and where I was headed. We agreed that the situation was not as perfectly good as we would have preferred, but it was not anywhere close to being as bad as it could have been. I told Eva that even if the tumor had been benign, the probability was that I would have had to submit to periodic exams through the coming years to make certain that I had not developed another one. So, as far as periodic checkups were concerned, my life had not changed upon Dr. Barnett's visit. True, his visit did change our perception of my tumor: It (the tumor) went from possibly wearing a white hat to definitely wearing a black one.

Nevertheless, it seemed we had run the bad guy out of town.

The future, I supposed, would take care of itself. There was no sense in worrying about it, and there arguably never is. I have often thought that the best way to prepare for the future is by taking care of business in the present. At present, there was still the business of the NG tube.

In a post surgery conversation I had with Dr. Leonard, he acknowledged that the current thinking among the newer members of the medical community is that this device is unnecessary for someone in my post surgical condition. Nonetheless, his expert experience insisted that I would have to suffer this apparatus' presence. In other words, the doc felt that the NG tube's possible benefit outweighed the inevitable torment that it would heap upon me. And the NG tube's presence becomes increasingly tormenting over time. Currently, it was hitting me with a one-two punch: terrible sore throat and raw left nostril. Anyone who has ever suffered this device knows what I am talking about. It's kind of like when people have the common experience of Catholic school attendance.

In spite of my deepening distress, Dr. Leonard had established that he would not permit the tube to be removed until I farted (his word) at least one time. He said that the event did not have to cause the walls to vibrate. A respectable toot would do. Normally, breaking wind is no problem for me, as my wife can attest. However, my whole digestive system had been completely emptied; the premises had been vacated. "So where was the gas to come from?" I wondered. I could have lied about meeting the criterion for the tube's removal, but I would not. Doing so might have been dangerously counterproductive and, almost as bad, in violation of my self-proclaimed policy of fully cooperating with those providing my treatment. Through Thursday, I had passed no gas. I was understandably becoming obsessed with generating just one expulsion. I remember thinking, "My kingdom for a fart." I even made this statement to Brian Holst during one of his visits following my surgery. As I recall, it took him by surprise.

Over three quarters of Friday had passed, but no gas. Being sympathetic, and perhaps empathetic in some of their cases, my attending nurses would regularly listen for sound in the area of my stomach and lower abdomen using a stethoscope. By this point, I could sometimes hear gastro-growls with the unaided ear, and feel them, too. All very encouraging, but I still could not produce.

On Friday, I redoubled my walking exercises, hoping to promote the occurrence of what I had come to call the "fortuitous flatulence." There were a couple of times during Friday afternoon that I thought the eventful venting would occur, but I was let down each time nothing was let out. Around six thirty Friday evening, Eva and I stood looking southward through my room's window. I watched various people traverse the parking lot as they traveled to and from the hospital. I thought them lucky in that probably all of them could pass gas effortlessly. Indeed, they might even have to fight the urge to do so, if they had found themselves in some social context that forbade this biological function, at least to any noticeable extent. "Lucky dogs," I thought. And then I suddenly felt a very welcomed pressure in my lower abdomen. This feeling was almost immediately followed by a very audible escape of gas.

At this much-anticipated moment, Eva was standing to my right.

Her nearly simultaneous and sharp turn of her head in my direction indicated that I was not suffering from an auditory hallucination. We both grinned with relief, mine greater than hers, in one another's direction, and then I commanded, "Get the nurse." I meant to be rid of the obnoxious tube immediately.

A male nurse named Scott happened to be on duty. I think that he was almost as relieved as I was that I had passed the necessary test allowing for the NG tube's removal. As Eva stood some distance at my left, Scott had me sit in a chair and removed the tape that was used to hold the tube semi-securely in my nostril. He advised that the only way to properly (i.e., with minimum pain) remove a NG tube is with great speed. He called this a "male thing." However, I cannot imagine that his tactic had application only in the case of males. Scott took his position in front of me, assuming a specific posture and gripping the end of the tube protruding from my nostril.

"Are you ready?" he asked.

"You bet, " I replied.

He yanked on the tube in a downward motion. It was gone from my anatomy in a flash. Nonetheless, I felt every millimeter of its length pass out of my body. And I mean *every* millimeter.

Now lighter by the weight of the tube, I sat stunned for maybe five seconds. I could not recall ever feeling so thoroughly and appreciatively liberated. The soreness in my throat was completely gone. My nose also felt much better. I took a brief look at my tormentor as Scott took it to the trash. It looked as ugly as it had felt. Good riddance!

During the June following my surgery, I attended a class concerning health maintenance. Much of the focus of the course was dietary. The instructor of the course used taped segments of the Oprah Winfrey Show to aid in instruction. During one such segment, a famous surgeon made mention that humans, both men and women, anally pass gas fourteen times per day. Yes, even women, which my wife vehemently denies. Personally, I thought this number erroneous on the low side. Anyway, I mentally chuckled while thinking, "Not so long ago, I could barely produce one blast in four days, let alone fourteen in one."

Well, a major hurdle was cleared in that fortuitous moment. I would have to clear two others in order to earn discharge from the hospital: peeing (after the catheter's removal) and pooping. Let it suffice to say that both of these hurdles were cleared with no difficulty. Thank God!

Once the tube was gone, I could eat. In fact, I would learn later that Dr. Leonard had given me carte blanche in this regard. This is to say that I could have called in a pizza, had I chosen and had I been able to tolerate it. The factor of toleration was one I would soon come to appreciate. Anyway, permission of an unrestricted menu had eluded me, and it seemed Eva, too. So, my first meal consisted of foods like bullion broth, gelatin, applesauce, sorbet, fruit juice and the like. I was thinking of asking for round two of my smorgasbord, when my stomach began to feel uneasy. Normally, the aforementioned foods would not give me any trouble, but my stomach was out of eating shape. I would have to be more cognizant of my stomach's sensitivity. It had been over eight days since I had eaten. Even the greatest of athletes, having been absent from the playing field, need a period of time to re-acclimate. And when it comes to eating, I am a great athlete!

Once my belly sent me the message to back off, I did. Before going to sleep that night, however, I would develop a craving for saltine crackers. Eva tracked down a supply in a break room on my floor and saw to it that I had several packets of crackers at my disposal before she parted for home that night. This fondness for saltines would stick with me for quite some time. In fact, a few sound real appetizing as I write!

All things considered, Friday the Thirteenth had not been too bad, not too bad at all. I went to sleep that night feeling more than a little lucky.

CHAPTER NINE

Saturday Night There'll Be No Fightin'

HROUGH **Friday, Eva** and I had successfully kept visitors to a manageable minimum. If not tightly managed, I feared the matter of receiving visitors would have gotten out of hand. I took few phone calls, as well. This is the way we agreed the matter of crowd control should be handled right from the beginning. And Eva took the agreement seriously, very seriously.

I feel compelled to mention that my insistence for social solitude was driven in large measure by my reluctance to be viewed like some animal in a zoo. This is a harsh description of how I viewed my relationship with visitors, I understand, but it's simply my nature to prefer the tranquility of solitude when I must lick my wounds, in a manner of speaking. Furthermore, I felt extremely frail and vulnerable, as mentioned before. People being physically around me made me nervous to the point of annoyance. For instance, a dear friend of mine about gave me a heart attack. As it was, she actually placed her left hand on my stomach area with the intention of supporting herself as she attempted to lean over my bed (and across my torso) to view a piece of equipment on my left. I arrested her intent before she could generate any significant pressure with her hand. Whew!

One permitted visitation was from the guys with whom I breakfast on Saturdays. Brian Holst, also a member of this breakfast club, had visited me, for both legal and personal reasons, more than anyone other than Eva. He remarked at about mid-week that it was getting harder and harder to keep the breakfast guys at bay. So, I gave the green light. I figured I owed this to my friends, and I also felt that seeing them would be good therapy for me, of a spiritual type. Eva concurred, but true to form, she insisted that the visit be short, around twenty minutes. She was vigilant in her time keeping, too. There were a few previous occasions when she politely expelled folks when their time had expired. In performing this function, Eva was so nice that instead of being offended at their expulsions, folks were practically apologizing for having intruded in the first place. That's my wife!

I woke up feeling pretty good, generally, on Saturday, but I did not feel that I should have any significant amount of breakfast until later in the morning. When the guys called from the restaurant to see if I wanted them to bring me some breakfast, I declined, although a dish from the Skillet Selections (a category of specialties on the menu) called The Gypsy posed a short lived temptation. Although I was still reveling in my divorce from the NG tube, my belly was still tender territory, and I thought it best I not celebrate with The Gypsy. Another indication that it would be prudent for me to exercise dietary caution occurred when a whiff of Eva's coffee did not arouse any interest on my part, quite atypically, I might add. So, I cautiously broke my fast by taking a few saltines, some gelatin and a few sips of hot tea. Any future adjustments in my diet would be based upon how well my stomach received these.

Before my visitors arrived, Eva and I had some time to discuss my medical status, as defined by my pathology report. During our conversation, I got the impression that Eva was a mite less comfortable with my medical status than I was. She simply did not like having the word cancer tied to the name Jim, her Jim. To be sure, I was not thrilled with this association either. But I think that it is easier, in some ways, to be the afflicted than it is to be the one who loves the afflicted. At a point in our conversation, Eva remarked that, "Things will never be the same." She was right. A fellow cancer patient said to me a few months after my release from LUH, "Cancer is a dirty word. It changes you." She was right, too.

By the conversation's end, we pledged to count our considerable blessings and soldier on or, as one of Eva's best employees is fond of saying, "Deal!" And speaking of blessings, we agreed that I had been lucky in a number of regards.

The lucky occurrences (or non-occurrences) we counted were: the tumor bled without bursting; the tumor's bleeding led to its being discovered before it had gotten very large and spread; a ten-thirty opening to see the doctor on the very day we called for an appointment was almost miraculous; Dr. Coff's being able to see me on a rushed basis was more good luck; and Dr. Coff's being able to get me into Dr. Leonard's hands was a blessing, big time.

More good luck was on its way, but we would have to wait a couple of days before learning of it.

At around nine-thirty, the breakfast boys showed up, Starbucks beverages still in some of their hands. Brian, Dale, David and Don comprised the troop. Bud was in Canada. Robert had been considered MIA for months, if not over a year. Just ahead of their arrival, my second breakfast had been delivered. I decided on some cream of wheat as the main dish with some equally innocuous side dishes and drinks. As I looked up from my serving tray, I could see that Eva had stalled the guys at the door so as to caution them that no one could be ill (infectious). I had to grin. Once she was satisfied that they were medically safe, Eva ushered the guys into my room, reminding them that the visit would have to be kept short. My friends made their entry looking somewhat like a group of second graders on a field trip, and who were entering the area of a museum display just after getting their look-but-don't-touch orders from their teacher. With the exception of Brian, this was the first time these men had seen me in my LUH digs.

"Hey, come on in, guys," I said hospitably, following with, "Nice to see you. Yes, very nice to see you all."

As they replied to my greeting, I could see that each of them studied me rather closely while taking their positions around the room. This observation applied to Brian as well. Brian, I expect, was comparing my present appearance with how I looked the previous time he had visited, examining me for evidence of progress. The others were making their assessments, too, but without the benefit of a baseline. I reciprocated. Each one looked to be in good spirits and sound health.

I continued to eat as we talked because I knew my company would not mind. Even though Brian had kept the guys abreast of my misadventure, I figured that they would appreciate a brief accounting of events from the protagonist himself. They, of course, were free to pose questions and make comments as I narrated my own story. Their two most common sentiments were that they thought I looked pretty good, considering what I had just been through, and that they found it hard to believe that I could have been so insidiously ill, in the first place. I did not think it my place to comment on the former sentiment, but I sure could concur on the latter. And I did!

I cannot remember how long my company visited, but they had not worn out their welcome by the time they left. Even though I had not received any official word, it was logical that I would be released from the hospital on the coming Monday, so I expressed sincere gratitude to this group of friends for visiting me this singular time during my hospitalization. Upon their departure, the room was very noticeably empty, in more ways than one.

Having these guys come by did help to put some more wind back into my sails. Furthermore, in the coming weeks I would become eager to be able to visit with them at our normal venue. Being able to resume my attendance at Saturday breakfasts would serve as a benchmark in my total recovery, although I would be reluctant to treat such attendance as an indication of a return to "the good old days." After all, I had become a cancer patient. My new normal could never look like my old normal, never. As the lady said, "It changes you."

Another big event on Saturday was my abandonment of the walker. By this time, I really did not need it for support, as I previously mentioned. Evidently, the young lady on duty as my therapist on Saturday also recognized that the walker had become superfluous, at least as far as its intended use was concerned.

Accordingly, she dictated that my walking exercises, of ever increasing frequency and distance, were to be henceforth performed without the walker. Even without the walker, however, my posture while walking remained bent in the forward direction, and at an angle that was not much less than that incurred when I had used the walker. Months later, stretching my abdominal area would still result in feelings that were certainly annoying, if not mildly painful. During my post-op visit with Dr. Leonard at the end of May, he informed me that I might feel various sensations around my belly resulting from the surgery for years.

Regarding my dietary prowess, my stomach seemed primed for real chow late Saturday morning. Pancakes and bacon suddenly sounded very appetizing. I ordered these, along with a double serving of orange juice. Suffice it to say that my first real breakfast since my admission to the hospital was well received by my innards.

The remainder of Saturday was uneventful, which was good, especially in the medical sense of the description. Like the previous few days, and quite some number to come, I spent the day getting used to life in the slow lane, although I did seem to be picking up speed, steadily.

CHAPTER TEN

Sunday Was the Last Time

SUNDAY, ALTHOUGH GENERALLY nondescript, did provide for an exceptional event in the form of a visit from one Mr. Gerry Savage. Gerry was a good friend of mine, and he had a very cordial relationship with Eva, too. Additionally, he was the only person whom I would describe as having been a mentor to me in my early years of teaching chemistry. Gerry was one of the most admirable men I have ever met.

I first met Gerry under very formal circumstances. He was a member of the interview team that decided to give me a crack at the recently vacated chemistry position at Skyline High School. In fact, other than one other person on that team, specifically the head principal, Gerry, being the chairman of the science department, had the greatest voice in my being hired. The only reason that I put the principal ahead of Gerry in my having been hired is because the principal was the only member of the team who possessed veto power. Consequently, he could have vetoed my being unanimously selected by Gerry and the other two persons on the team simply because he did not like the gap between my top, middle, front teeth. A principal is a powerful force in his or her school. As someone once put it to me, "If a principal wants you, you're in; if he doesn't, you're out."

Gerry had been by to visit me on Thursday of the previous week, and he had been typically very talkative that day. And to his credit, Gerry could be very informative and entertaining on a number of different levels. In fact, he could be very entertainingly educational. But the truth is he stayed a bit too long that day. At that time, I was enduring a severe pummeling at the hands of the NG tube, and I was kind of beaten up generally. Nonetheless, I could not tell Gerry it was time for him to leave. It would almost have been like my telling my father that he had worn out his welcome. Eva, however, was not bound by any such constraint. Seeing that I was starting to visibly weaken, she announced that visitation hours had expired. Appreciating that Eva had my best interests in mind, Gerry complied with her announcement without delay or complaint. In only moments following her decree, Gerry was in Eva's escort and bound for points beyond my door. On Saturday, he called Eva on her cell phone to inquire about the acceptability of his visiting on Sunday, in the early afternoon after church, specifically. Eva granted permission, provided that the visit would be of short duration. Gerry understood, and he quickly consented to her condition regarding the visit's allowable length.

At around one o'clock Sunday, Gerry peered into my room and asked if it was permissible to enter. We quickly answered in the affirmative, and Gerry took the same seat he favored on his previous visit. I had never before seen him in a coat and tie, but I had never before seen him recently departed from church, either.

"I can't say that I ever saw you so spiffed up," I said while smiling broadly and laughing lightly.

Gerry came back with, "You look a lot better today, yourself."

"Yeah, life's a lot more enjoyable without a loathsome NG tube," was how I accounted for my improved appearance and, especially, improved spirits.

Gerry conveyed his understanding by chuckling while nodding.

Gerry possessed many qualities that would justify my calling him admirable. For example, he was gentlemanly, knowledgeable, considerate and honest, to mention just a few. But the quality of being helpful was Gerry's one quality I consider preeminent among the rest. To further this point, I call attention to Gerry's helpfulness at school. Whether the problem was in the form of a stubborn VCR, a complicated lab setup or a difficult calculation, Gerry always made himself available to assist the needy, if not frantic, teacher. His helpful nature was so well known that he was always the person other teachers in the math and science departments first sought for help. He was just as agreeable, furthermore, to helping *any* Skyline staff member. Lending a helping hand was so natural to Gerry that he even helped staff members whose presence he did not especially relish. I am sure that from Gerry's point of view, such folks qualified for receiving help simply because they were people in need. Gerry could no more deny a person in need than he could a student in need, personalities being without bearing.

I informed Gerry about the knowledge of my pathology report, knowledge that I did not have at the time of his previous visit. Gerry voiced concern about the matter of malignancy, but also optimism about my recovery, given the report's favorable data, overall. And being that Gerry knew me well, he took pains to caution me about the necessity to exercise patience with myself during my recovery. Of course, he made it clear to call him if I needed anything, anything at all. I thanked my old mentor and expressed agreement with his advice to take things easy, promising, for emphasis, to refrain from cutting down any trees in the near future. My promise was a thinly disguised reference to a favor Gerry had performed the previous day. True to form, Gerry had helped a friend by felling and removing a dead tree that had become a danger to his friend's residence. Since this person had no fireplace, Gerry loaded the cuttings into the bed of his nineteen sixty-five Ford pickup truck. His intention was to deliver the logs of his labors to someone who would have use for the firewood. He would expect no payment for any of this, to be sure, certainly nothing beyond the offer of a cup of coffee.

Honoring his agreement with Eva, Gerry kept his visit to an agreeable length. As he stood to excuse himself and shake hands, we promised one another that we would meet for breakfast as soon as my condition would permit. Such meetings were how we made sure to remain in touch once Gerry retired from teaching. And we would meet, pursuant to this objective, several times a year at one of his favorite greasy spoons. We also expressed intent to go out for a good dinner with the girls, his Sandra and my Eva. Eva enthusiastically concurred. The date was broadly selected as some time toward the end of June. I am sure Gerry had some witticism to leave me with as he departed because it was part of his style. Unfortunately, I cannot recall what it was.

The weather was very nice that Sunday, unlike the previous Sunday, Easter. A time or two earlier in the day, Eva and I had walked to my room's window to enjoy the view of the nicest spring day we had had to date. We decided to take another gander at nature's springtime display, and positioned ourselves at my room's window, which allowed for southward views. Gerry had parked his truck, logs and all, in a spot that was impossible to miss looking out this window. As soon as I saw the truck, I had to grin and call Eva's attention to it. Given the newness of the other vehicles in the vicinity of Gerry's truck, it looked humorously out of place, something like a laden mule would look hitched among a row of thoroughbreds. Seeing the truck meant that Gerry should soon be coming into our range of view. Sure enough, a few moments later we watched Gerry proceed through the crosswalk and into the lot as he made his way toward his truck. Gerry was a big guy who walked with a gait that reminded me of James Arness and John Wayne. His manner of walking was not identical to either man's, but contained components of both. We watched Gerry as he neared and, ultimately, entered his truck. He cranked the engine, causing his old mule to noticeably shudder, and then he began to urge it backward out of its stall. Once properly aligned in the lot's traffic lane, Gerry and his mount sauntered toward the west exit of the parking lot.

Sunday was the last time we would ever see Gerry.

He was the one in "ten thousand" to whom I made reference in a previous chapter.

Life being what it is, Eva and I had no way of knowing Gerry's fate. Accordingly, we continued onward through Sunday in high spirits. For one thing, I was eating normally again. In fact, my personal menu had expanded to include turkey sandwiches covered with gravy and accompanied by a side of mashed potatoes. Furthermore, I had been freed from the catheter earlier in the day, and I was urinating without any problems, very good news. Another cause for our high spirits was that I was having no problems with bowel movements. Being able to thus eliminate waste were two important conditions that had to be met before I could be discharged. Therefore, we had every reason to expect that I would be released from the hospital on Monday and, hopefully, earlier than later.

Another mark that indicated that I was making progress was my re-born interest in reading the newspaper, for myself, that is. I turned the television on for the first time in days, too. I had watched no TV since early Easter Sunday morning. The classic movie *Boys Town* happened to be on that morning, so I watched it for a distraction and the possibility of gaining some modicum of strength or inspiration from it. After Gerry left, I found some NBA games to half-heartedly watch as I read the Sunday paper. That evening, Eva and I watched another movie classic, this one from the fifties and starring Gregory Peck and Richard Basehart, *Moby Dick*.

I went to sleep that night feeling that although it would be a while before I was out of the woods, it was, nonetheless, time that I was out of the hospital.

CHAPTER ELEVEN

Goin' Home I'm Dreamin'

"**I**'M GOING HOME**,** today," was the thought I awoke with on Monday the sixteenth.

Logically, it seemed to me that four medical events had to occur before I could be legitimately discharged from LUH. First, I had to get the CAT-scan of my lungs that Dr. Barnett had ordered. Second, I had to meet with Dr. Barnett so that Eva and I could learn of his checkup plan for me. Third, Dr. Leonard would have to give his consent for my release after examining me. Fourth, I would have to have the staples removed from my incision. The last event was the one about which I was least certain. Perhaps the staples would come out at a later date. Anyway, none of these appeared to present a serious impediment to my escape.

Eva arrived just ahead of eight o'clock, only minutes before I was taken to the CAT-scan room. She was pleased at her timeliness because it permitted her to accompany me to my scanning session. We both greeted my driver as he steered an empty chair into my room. In mere moments after his arrival, I was seated and being wheeled to my appointment. Eva kept pace even though it appeared my driver had had a high-octane breakfast.

A lung scan does not require the patient to consume any sort of foul mixture or solution, and the actual scan is a piece of cake. Immediately after the scan was performed, I was whisked back to my room, much to my liking because I was marking time. Although lacking the hospital's imprimatur, my timetable would hold if I were back in my room before either doctor showed up.

As I had hoped, the speedy return to my room was "just what the doctor ordered." I barely had time to use the bathroom and resettle into my bed before Dr. Barnett showed up, and well ahead of nine o'clock. His having shown up so early bolstered my confidence that I would be leaving soon because Dr. Leonard's track record indicated that he would be in for an early visit, too.

After the three of us exchanged greetings, and the doc made inquiry as to how I was feeling, he seated himself in a chair near the foot of my bed. Doc appeared to be in high spirits, a bit excited, in fact.

Dr. Barnett's early visit meant that he had not had the time to see my scan images. As it was, he would have to report his interpretation of the scan's images at a later date, perhaps when I made my first visit to his office or by telephone. He assured me he suspected nothing wrong with my lungs. He just needed a starting set of images for the sake of reference.

The doc did have news of another sort, however. He wanted to change the plan for my post-operative life. Eva and I were, of course, very interested in the nature of the change and the reasoning behind it. The doctor went on to explain.

As I understand things, Dr. Barnett was surfing the net during the night of the Friday on which he had earlier first visited me in the afternoon. In so doing, he came upon the results of a clinical trial that had just been made available to the public during the previous day, Thursday the twelfth. The trial involved a very large number of GIST patients, was sponsored by the National Cancer Institute, and was conducted by a network of researchers. The trial's good news for me is as follows: "Researchers found that approximately 97 percent of patients in the study who received one year of imatinib mesylate (Gleevec) after surgery did not have a recurrence of their cancer compared to 83 percent of patients who received one year of placebo."

Before knowing the results of this trial, the doctor would not have recommended I take Gleevec. Indeed, at the time of our first meeting, Dr. Barnett was of the opinion that a follow up drug therapy was, in a case like mine, without merit. GIST tumors, by the way, are notoriously indifferent to chemo and radiation therapy. Gleevec is not a form of chemotherapy, as I will explain soon.

"Well, this is interesting," I thought, and in some form or another, I am betting that Eva did, too.

Had all that had happened to me occurred in exactly the same way two years earlier, for example, I would have been sent home after surgery with no further treatment and with an eighty-three percent chance of non-recurrence. So, this *was* big news for me, and it would add to the series of lucky breaks Eva and I enumerated on Saturday. Understandably, I was eager to capitalize on my additional good fortune.

"Sign me up, Doc. I'm game," was my immediate reply to the doc's suggestion that I get on board with Gleevec for a year.

Dr. Barnett acknowledged my prudent decision and promised to get me going with the Gleevec in about a month. The delay was necessary to give me time to regain my strength. Although Gleevec is additionally appealing because of patients' low incidences of intolerable side effects, it can, nonetheless, produce some serious ones. As my strength improved, so did my chances of being able to tolerate the drug.

Dr. Barnett also explained that Gleevec is a "targeted therapy," and targeted therapy is not a program of chemotherapy. In Dr. Barnett's words, "Chemotherapy is like a carpet bombing campaign. Targeted therapy is like using a smart bomb."

"Better living through chemistry, huh, Doc?" I offered.

He laughed.

I also want to mention that not too long after being released from the hospital, I learned that a delayed effect of some type (or types) of chemotherapy could be the development of at least one type of leukemia. Hair loss during chemotherapy would have been of zero concern to me. Leukemia, on the other hand, is a horse of a very different color.

Before leaving, Dr. Barnett asked when I thought I would be going home. I told him I hoped it would be sometime that morning. Knowing that he would likely not see me again before I left the hospital, the doc made sure I knew how to get in touch with his office, and we settled on a date for my first office visit.

We thanked Dr. Barnett for his time and efforts. He assured us that he was as delighted to be able to deliver such good news as we were to receive it, and then he took his leave of us.

Eva and I were abuzz about the targeted therapy. "Fourteen percentage points" became our new favorite phrase.

I have for many years appreciated that we all endure the element of risk as we live a life buffeted by chance. My guess is that somewhere around adolescence, most people become mindful of the uncertain nature of life. Nonetheless, we march on, each individual subconsciously hopeful that the odds gods are smiling on him or her at any given moment in the march. In this time of medical crisis, however, Eva and I had become acutely conscious of, if not preoccupied with, the odds, especially those prognosticated by the medical odds-makers.

The man arguably most responsible for improving my odds, namely, Dr. John Leonard, charged into my room, in his typical man-on-a-mission manner, not long after Dr. Barnett had gone. Dr. Leonard's arrival came close enough to Dr. Barnett's departure that I asked if the two had bumped into one another somewhere on the west fourth floor. They had not. Anyway, events were flowing so favorably that it seemed that I had choreographed them. Dr. Leonard's timely arrival allowed me to speculate that the time remaining before my discharge from LUH would be under an hour. At this point, I could not imagine Dr. Leonard would find any reason to extend my hospitalization. I was correct.

The doc led with, "How are you doing?"

"Fine," I answered, quickly following with, "Real good, Doc," intending to imply that I was sufficiently recovered (and expecting) to go home.

"What did Dr. Barnett have to say this morning?"

While I recounted the particulars of Dr. Barnett's visit, Dr. Leonard listened intently and approvingly. I think that the doctor expected and *wanted* to hear a report of a rigorous and vigilant post-operative plan for the continuance of my fight against cancer. Two points would seem to support this contention. First, Dr. Leonard had highly recommended Dr. Barnett, indicating they have a similar view of what constitutes the best treatment for a post-operative cancer patient. Second, some weeks later during one of my visits to Dr. Leonard's office, the doctor made certain to make the point that I was "not to allow myself to fall through the cracks." My interpretation of this advice is: Never allow the system to forget about me; be a pest, if necessary, but be sure that all is being done to win my fight against cancer. In other words, I was to insist on rigorousness and vigilance in my future treatment. I, of course, intend to follow this advice religiously because, for one reason, it just makes good sense. For another reason, Eva was in the office, and she heard the doctor's every word, too!

When it was obvious that I was nearing the end of the details of the Barnett plan, Doc approached my bed indicating that he wanted to inspect my incision. Although it had been almost seven full days since my surgery, I still had not really looked at my forming scar. When the doc removed the gauze covering my incision this time, he did so with no intention of reaffixing it to my abdomen. From this point forward, I would have no need of a gauze covering. I did not look much at the scar this time either, choosing to study the doc's face to deduce my state of healing. The quickness of the exam and the look of impassiveness on the doc's face allowed me to know the incision appeared as the doc expected.

"Good," I thought.

"I'll get someone in here to get those staples out. Once they're out, you can be on your way home," the doc announced.

"Dang," I thought.

Of course, I liked the part about going home, but I was hoping to delay the inevitability of the staples' removal for some other day. There always seems to be a price to pay. Staple removal would be the voucher du jour.

No longer concerned with my cut, Doc applied his attention to the pain ball.

Unlike the staples, the doc saw fit to remove this apparatus, himself. In the process of doing so, he indicated that the ball was empty. Interesting. I had no idea that the ball was dry. This state of ignorance allowed me to reason that I was healing rather painlessly and, therefore, properly. From this point forward, I would only take Vicodin for pain, and only when I thought it necessary to do so. And I would not think it necessary to pop a Vicodin very often. As I write this paragraph, nearly four months after my release from the hospital, about sixteen pills (a third of the original and only prescription) remain in the pharmacy issued bottle. By calling attention to my limited need of the Vicodin prescription, I only hope to acknowledge the terrific job Dr. Leonard did in taking me apart and then putting me back together again. My limited use of the pain pills has nothing to do with my toughness. I assure all that had I been in any real pain, I would have polished off the bottle in short order!

I would guess that the pain ball apparatus, once exhausted of its chemical magic, would qualify as little more than trash. However, I cannot recall Dr. Leonard dropping the spent apparatus into the trashcan near my bed, although he must have done so. Because my relationship with the pain ball was entirely different from that with the NG tube, perhaps I did not feel compelled to derive some satisfaction in witnessing its discard and, consequently, made no effort to mark the event.

The anesthesiologist had removed the epidural the previous night. The process was as quick and painless as that of the pain ball's removal.

It seemed prudent to check with Doc about what I would and would not be permitted to do when I was once again home. So, even before he had completely finished removing the pain ball, I asked, "What are the do's and don'ts when I get home, Doc?"

As he was wrapping up his work with the ball, Dr. Leonard replied, but without looking at me, "You can do anything you want." Then after a brief pause, he followed with the caveat, "Within reason."

I was silent, a bit perplexed by his answer.

The doc had probably gotten the response he wanted. By this I mean to say that Dr. Leonard, in my experience, enjoys giving a simple answer when, perhaps, one is expecting a response that is more complicated, or even ornate. I, for one, appreciate his policy of keeping things as simple as possible for his patients. What could possibly be a better policy?

Now finished with all of his duties relative to my incision and pain ball, the doc positioned himself so as to look me in the eyes. He then deciphered his answer.

"Reasonable daily living," he began, "must become the guiding principle in your recovery." "Of course," he quickly added, "what reasonable daily living looks like will change from day-to-day, as you develop momentum in your recovery."

Dr. Leonard liked to use scientific terminology, such as momentum, when we conversed. I took this as a compliment.

I logically concluded that reasonable daily living covered sex, too, so I next launched a question about diet.

"How about eating?" I continued, seeking mostly a reply that would confirm, as opposed to inform, since I had been allowed an unrestricted diet upon the NG tube's removal.

"Unrestricted. Have anything you want. Just don't over eat. Do a lot of grazing," he replied, in staccato style.

I took the advice about overeating to heart. Although my digestive system seemed to be working miraculously well, at least from the point of view of a layman like me, I figured things still had to be a bit tender and unsettled in those regions. I sure did not want to cause myself trouble by excessively taxing my digestive machinery, especially my small intestine.

The doc would later construct some impressive imagery regarding my diet. This construction would occur during the office visit he had me schedule for Thursday of that week. During the visit, his imaginative advice for my diet was, "Eat lots of meat and potatoes, good Yankee food." He then went on to say, "Protein will be the bricks, and sugar will be the mortar, of your reconstruction." Eva was present when the doc said this. The menu at the Gaudio residence reflected for weeks her intention to make me a masonry masterpiece.

His work in room 4006 done for the day, at least as far as I was concerned, the doc took his leave, but not before assuring us that someone would soon be in to pull my staples.

Now that I had been officially cleared for departure, Eva started to earnestly pack my things and to ready them for transport. I would describe her at this time as being equally nervous and excited about my return home. These psychological states clearly energized her, making her movements humorously accelerated.

As advertised, a nurse arrived within minutes of Dr. Leonard's exit, and she had a sidekick with her. I recognized the RN because she had tended to me once before, but her assistant was entirely new to me. Also, when I was introduced to the woman working under the RN's direction, I came to the erroneous conclusion that she was a student engaged in some sort of nursing practicum.

After a brief session of polite chitchat that mostly concerned my imminent trip home, these women disconnected me from the IV tree and freed me from the IV needle, as well. Next, the nurse informed me that the staples would be removed as soon as they returned with the necessary tools with which to do the job. Both women looked at my cut in order to assure they would be properly equipped to pull the staples upon their return. As for me, I still had not yet given the incision a bona fide visual inspection.

Before leaving, they assured me that they would not be gone long, understanding that I would not want my escape to be unnecessarily delayed. In watching them depart, it was my expectation that the RN would do the staple pulling.

True to their word, the women soon returned with a set of staple pulling tools. As I lay in my bed, the nurse's assistant instructed me to arrange my gown and blankets in such a way as to make my incision accessible. She then laid out the staple pulling tools along a lengthwise folded towel running parallel to my right leg. It looked to me like the assistant was doing a nice job of getting things ready for the RN to pull the staples. I was wrong.

When she was satisfied that all was ready, the assistant picked up one of the tools, looked at me and, to my considerable surprise, asked, "Are you ready?"

"You're pulling the staples?" I replied with a tone indicating concern.

"Yes," the assistant answered, obviously caught off guard by my doubt regarding her abilities.

Without intending to insult the woman, who was probably in her forty's, I responded to her affirmation with, "But aren't you just a nursing student? Do you have any experience doing this sort of thing?"

With a wide smile and shaking her head slightly she answered, "Oh, no. I've been a LPN for years. I've done this many times."

Seeking clarification, I said, "But I thought you said you're a student."

"I am. I'm working toward becoming a registered nurse."

I felt a little embarrassed, but she was obviously amused, saving me from feeling too stupid. But I still felt compelled to apologize.

"I'm sorry. I misunderstood."

She consoled me with, "No problem."

"Well, I guess we might as well get started," I suggested, feeling that I was as ready for this procedure as I would ever be.

"OK."

I figured that the point along the cut at which she would start pulling staples was probably more a matter of preference than science. So, when she started her work at the top staple, I saw no reason to question her decision, either mentally or audibly.

It was during the staples' removal that I looked at my incision for the first time. And I mean that I *really* looked at it, staple by staple. As the crow flies, the scar measures seven inches. Its total track, however, is somewhat longer because the scar resembles an elongated letter s, due to the surgeon's need to veer around my bellybutton as he cut.

So, being that there were probably more that twenty staples, I had a good, long first look at my forming scar. The staples measured, I approximated, a quarter inch wide and equally long. To be sure, they were substantial entities; otherwise they could not be trusted to keep the incision securely closed. However, their removal was not as painful as it may have appeared. Nonetheless, I was eager to get this matter behind me.

The LPN was doing a fine job. I was clearly in capable hands. Things were proceeding swimmingly until she got about two-thirds down the cut. At this point, she encountered a staple that wanted to be uncooperative about its removal.

"Figures," I mentally complained. I also hoped that this would be the only devil among the group. It was not.

After unsuccessfully struggling with the uncooperative staple for perhaps thirty seconds, the assistant decided to skip it and to go back for it later. Downward she continued, but at a point a couple of staples further along, she ran into another staple that was reluctant to give up its residence in my skin.

"Terrific," I disgustedly said under my breath, upset with my deteriorating luck, not the LPN.

Again, she chose to skip over the uncooperative staple. Luckily, the remaining staples gave up without much of a fight. Back she went to get the troublemakers.

I should note that this woman talked to me all the while she was working. In particular, she would routinely ask how I was doing. I do not think that I orally answered this question even once. Instead, I would only nod my response while offering a weak smile. This was the politest way I knew to urge the assistant along without my being pushy. I think it was effective.

Posthaste, she returned to the second of the two offending staples. Surprisingly, it came out without too much coaxing this time around. The LPN voiced pleasure at this staple's removal without offering any explanation for its suddenly becoming cooperative.

Finally, she returned to the first offender. This staple's attitude had not changed appreciably since the practical nurse's first attempt to extract it. So the LPN chose, for the first time, to try using another of the several tools she had previously laid on the towel. Unfortunately for me, even the new tool could not convince this obnoxious staple to play ball.

The RN remained silently standing near my left, observing, but evidently unconcerned.

The assistant showed some frustration over this staple's stubbornness, but I could see that she remained confident. The tone of her voice remained calm and controlled, as she now talked more to the staple than to me. She continued to angle this way and that with the metallic tool she wielded in her right hand. In the absence of any indication, at least as far as I could tell, the staple suddenly yielded to the force of the assistant's effort, and it bid me farewell, so to speak. I bid it something, too, so to speak.

"Done," I said to myself. I then sincerely congratulated the LPN on the nice job she did. She smiled her reply, almost as if to say, "I told you that I know what I'm doing."

The RN now became actively involved in what might be considered the mopping up portion of the job. Both women participated in cleaning my incision and the area around it. They, as did Dr. Leonard, commented that the wound looked good, in the sense that it appeared to be properly healing. And as the doctor had done, they noted that my skin does not particularly cotton to a certain type of medical tape the hospital uses to secure various items to a patient's body. I had several nasty blisters from this tape, and the nurses attended to these using some sort of ointment and then a covering of gauze. They used a paper tape to secure the gauze, and advised I follow suit in the future. I still sport noticeable scars from big blisters caused by the other type of tape.

The last work these women did on my incision was to apply quite a number of adhesive strips along it. These strips looked like anti-snoring nasal strips, and they were placed across my incision and perpendicular to it. By the time the last strip was on, the combination of my incision and the strips looked similar to the threaded area on a football. The purpose of these strips was to help to keep the incision pulled together. I did not say anything to the nurses, but I guessed that Dr. Leonard would scoff at these strips when he saw them on Thursday. Judging from what I knew of the man, I had to believe he would look at the nurses' work as being without medical merit. I was right. When he saw me on Thursday, the first words out of his mouth when he saw the incision were, "Who did this?" I honestly answered, "The nurses who pulled my staples." The doc then shook his head disapprovingly while commenting, "Once something gets into the medical lexicon, it's virtually impossible to get it out." Such strips, of course, would not visit my incision again.

I should not fail to mention that during the above-mentioned visit to Dr. Leonard's office, he bushwhacked me with one heck of a surprise. While examining my incision, he took into hand a cotton swab of the medical variety. Unlike a Q-tip, this construction consisted of a single cotton swab that was wound around the end of a thin stick about six inches long. The stick's diameter was slightly greater than that of a round style toothpick at its midpoint. With swab in hand, the doc called Eva over to the examination table on which I lay, my incision fully exposed. Then, and with no warning, the doc plunged the swab into my incision at a point about three inches below my bellybutton.

"This is how you drain the incision, nurse Gaudio," he informed Eva.

He had buried the full length of the swab into my cut and was swirling it clockwise and counterclockwise as he held the stick between an index finger and thumb. Eva was stunned and made nauseous by this act to the point that she had to resume her seat. As Dr. Leonard finished up with this draining procedure, he told Eva that she would have to do this once per day, for a week. Eva is tough when she has to be, and she would have done her duty, like it or not. However, I had made up my mind on the spot that it was my incision, so it would be my duty to drain it. With the use of a hand-held mirror, I would perform the procedure at the same point along the cut that the doc had, and I would do so for seven consecutive days. As would be expected, the force necessary to push the swab into my incision increased as the cut healed a little more each day. Nevertheless, the matter *looked* more painful than it was, much like the pulling of the staples.

Having finished with all their work relative to my staples, the RN and LPN took their leave of me, promising to promptly have an attendant with a wheelchair in my room and to provide any further assistance I might need in effecting my exit. It was still less than an hour since Dr. Leonard had left, and I was apparently mere minutes away from "getting out of Dodge."

Getting me into street clothes now became the newest task. With Eva's help, I was dressed in a flash, and a good thing, too, because the attendant with the wheelchair was at the door just after I had finished getting my shoes on. Eva had to assist me with my shoes this time, but never thereafter. A little footstool we have at home allowed me to avoid excessive bending when putting on my shoes.

Once again, I was perfectly capable of walking, but hospital policy insisted that I be transported from my room to the hospital's main entrance (the entrance nearest where Eva had parked) via a wheelchair. As stated previously, I do not relish riding in one of these contraptions. I find the experience to be intimidating. I think that I view the need of a wheelchair as a form of incarceration. How a person deals with such confinement for life I truly cannot fathom. Yet I am forced to acknowledge that, until just recently, I could not fathom dealing with cancer, either.

Anyway, in what I hope was my last wheelchair ride, I was forced to suffer the indignity of the ridiculous. As it was, there was some reason that the attendant showed up at my room with a wheelchair that is designed to transport folks of a size comparable to that of the larger among those who count themselves as offensive tackles in the NFL. When I took my seat in that chair, I looked as much undersized as I would have had I attempted to wear the uniform of one of the aforementioned football players. I could not even place my feet on the rests that allow the rider to keep his or her feet comfortably positioned during transport. Furthermore, the lady attendant had a very difficult time commanding this vehicle to move in a desired direction. I could not wait to get out of this oversized wheelchair and into the comfortable seating of my wife's car.

Wanting to remain true to my intent to cooperate fully with those who were responsible for my care, I decided to endure, one last time. In fact, I think I did a little better than simply enduring. To be sure, nobody would have mistaken me for some politician riding in a parade. Nevertheless, upon seating myself in this cavernous chair, I rolled down the hallway with a wide smile, waving thank you and fond farewell to those who had cared for me both directly and indirectly. Had I really been on the ball, I would have tossed some of my lemon drops to my adoring crowd. I am confident, however, that these good folks much more enjoyed the cheesecake and sliced strawberries (in lots of berry juice) that Eva and I delivered to them some weeks later.

Once at the end of the hall, I found myself positioned in front of the public-use elevators. Eva, of course, had been at my side or in my wake all along our routing. Not one to be left out, she had a wheeled vehicle, too. The nurses who last attended me saw that Eva had much too much stuff to tote in her arms, so they secured a cart for her convenience. Without this cart, Eva would have had to make at least two separate trips to get all of our things from room 4006 to her car.

An elevator's doors finally opened, and the attendant managed to get me into the elevator's car, but only through a considerable expenditure of her energy. At least that is how it sounded from where I sat. Without doubt, Eva's entry was much more fluid. It was a good thing that no other people wanted to board the elevator with us because space in its car was definitely at a premium. We descended.

As soon as the elevator's doors opened sufficiently, we could see that the lobby was busy with various people on sundry missions. This mix of people included, to my best estimation, hospital employees, delivery people, patients and visitors. To my already taxed attendant, the lobby must have appeared to be a veritable obstacle course. I could not imagine she felt otherwise, based upon my ride to this point.

"This ought to be interesting," I thought as I surveyed the potential impediments, human and other, that lay between the elevators and the area beyond the automatic doors where I would wait for Eva to bring her car around. While being pushed across the lobby, I would be akin to a pinball trying to find its way past moving obstacles, instead of stationary ones. The possibilities for collisions between the pinball (me) and some obstacle, human or inanimate, were limited only by one's imagination. And I was concerned about being involved in a collision for two reasons, one emotional and the other physical. Emotionally, I simply did not need any hassle in completing the final leg of my exit. Period. Physically, I knew that I was frail, and felt so. Consequently, I found the thought of being bumped to any extent to be positively frightful.

I had underestimated my attendant. She evidently is the type who performs best under pressure. I came to this conclusion because, and much to my delight, she required a minimal amount of time and energy to deftly steer me through all of the commotion and onto the walkway where I would remain parked until Eva came around in her car. We were so quickly through the lobby, I must add, that an acquaintance from church that I had spied to our right did not have an opportunity to catch sight of us. Good! I was in no mood for small talk or for answering any questions.

Once outside, Eva parked her handcart next to me, then she made a dash for her car. The attendant stood at my right, somewhat like a guard. The weather was damp and cool. The air not only felt good, but it smelled good, in spite of all the cars and smokers in this canopied, drive-up area. I remember thinking that it felt good to be homeward bound, but strange, too. My stay at LUH was like passing through a portal into a different life, a strange life, the life of a cancer patient.

My wife is a heck of a good driver. Well, of course she is: I was her driving instructor! Within moments of her departure, Eva had negotiated her Accord into just the right parking space to load me. Despite all the traffic, both wheeled and pedestrian, Eva was the personification of fluidity. The car now parked, Eva came around its rear and ordered, "OK. Let's get you in."

With practically no help at all, I vacated the wheelchair and seated myself in the front passenger seat. As the attendant was just beginning to retreat with the oversized wheelchair, and just before Eva closed the car's door, I thanked my wheelchair pusher for her help. It only took Eva a few moments to complete loading the car. When done loading, she scurried around to the driver's side of the car and hopped in. Once seated, she strapped herself in and checked that I had done so, too. Then we were on our way. It had not yet been an hour since Dr. Leonard had given me the green light to go home.

"I'm alive. At least I'm leaving the hospital, *alive*," I thought.

We made the short drive home in only minutes, and in a very

light rain that required the wipers to only intermittently attend the windshield. As we pulled into the driveway, Eva pressed the button on the remote control for the garage door opener. By the time she had stopped the car and came around to open my door, the garage door was completely open, allowing an unimpeded view into our two-car garage. With considerably more difficulty than when I had gotten into the car, I got out, and then I moved away from the car's door so that I would not be in the way of its closing. In the process of distancing myself from the car, I had become positioned on the driveway such that I found myself looking directly into my garage. I refer to the garage as being "mine" because it is. The only time Eva is in the garage is when she is doing one of the following: parking or removing her car; or searching for some item believed in her car; or putting something into or taking something out of the freezer; or looking for some gardening tool or fertilizer or insecticide. I, on the other hand, can spend hours at a time in the garage. In the course of a typical week, I can easily spend eight hours in *my* garage.

One of the thoughts I had while hospitalized was whether I would ever again see *my* garage. Grappling with cancer has a profound effect on one's thinking.

CHAPTER TWELVE

Bare Naked Thoughts

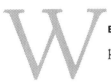**ELL, SO HERE** I am, a member of the cancer patients' club.

Who would have thought?

Not I.

But once I became a club member, or even suspected that I would be, a lot of thoughts flowed through my mind. What follows is a display of some of those thoughts. They are presented in no particular order or grouping. I simply went with the flow, as we say, and without any intention to preach to anyone, to lecture to anyone or to convert anyone.

Like most people, I suspect, I have given no small amount of thought to death over the course of my life. About fifteen years ago, I finally developed a theological position about the inevitability of my death that I could *live* with. In my hour of trial, however, death moved out of my peripheral vision and into a more direct line of sight. The question then became whether or not I could *die* with my theology. And this is exactly what I thought to myself while being wheeled downstairs to surgery. Specifically, I honestly asked myself if I thought I needed to make any last minute adjustments regarding my theological views. I did not. I felt that my way of thinking was an honest and sensible response to the mysteries not one of us has figured out, or ever will. My manner of prayer remained unchanged at the hour during which I most needed to pray.

Another thought that I suppose was inevitable was, "Why me?" The answer to this question, in my view, is, "Why not me?" For a long, long time, now, I have been of the philosophical position that life is a crapshoot. Tough luck happens to people every minute of every day. That is just the way it is. Period. So, the answer to, "Why me?" had to be, "Why not me?" I am, after all, nobody special.

Besides the element of fright, the prospect of death held for me an element of annoyance, as well. The cause of this annoyance was the odious thought of my dying while Eva is still alive. In short, I hated (and hate) the thought of having to give up the girl. Selfish? Sure! But I do not care. My feelings ran so deep in this matter that I would at times imagine myself dead, but able to look in on Eva. In such a thought experiment, as Einstein might have called it, I would see her, for example, eating at the kitchen table. I could feel her heart ache as she noted the permanent absence of a place setting for me. This type of thought, more than any other, brought me closest to tears.

As regards tears, I thought a few times that perhaps I should just break down and cry. But then I would think that crying would solve nothing. If the act of producing tears could have set everything right, I would have cried two rivers, one from each eye.

I thought about how I always worried about Boots' health and safety, especially as she advanced in age. Mostly when I was yet in the hospital, I thought of how ironic it would be if I were to precede Boots in death. As it came to be, however, our much-loved Boots did not survive me. I had to euthanize her less than three months after my return home.

On numerous occasions I thought of how a patient might not want to go on living in the absence of someone for whom to live, the absence of someone who *wanted* the patient to live. It is not my intention to imply that my recent ordeal, minus my loving Eva, would have found me refusing medical attention and simply crawling under the covers to await death. Instead, I am saying that without Eva, I would have been much, much more indifferent about the outcome of my medical misadventure. It is now little wonder to me that a surviving spouse of a long-time couple sometimes dies soon after the death of his or her life-partner. I certainly did draw strength from the prayers and well wishes of others, as I previously acknowledged. But nothing inspired me to want to win my fight, as did Eva, my raison d'etre. Almost as soon as we learned that I had a tumor, my wife established a beacon by which we could navigate our way through our travail. "It's us," she declared, meaning, "It's all about us." We were, by her edict, to never allow ourselves to lose sight of the singular objective to arrive at the other end of this trauma a couple. And Eva would accept nothing short of my living up to my end of the bargain.

Sometimes I think, "A GIST. Of all the damn things! I can't believe it. I just can't believe it."

Having cancer is like jousting with the devil, although I view my joust with the beast an easy one, relative to that of some folks, at least so far. In this combat, I feared I would be cowardly. Cowardly behavior always worries me. The last thing I wanted was to fall apart, becoming a blubbering emotional wreck, profoundly embarrassing myself in my wife's presence and causing her even more distress. I wanted to impress my wife, not depress her. I think it would be better to die than to pathetically falter.

My fear of cowardice (failure) made me wonder more than once if I could handle going through all of this (or worse) again. I just do not know, and I try to avoid thinking about it. I sincerely hope that fate does not demand an encore.

Facing the chance that my life could soon be over caused me to think about teaching in the public schools. To the point, I wondered if such employment was an unjustifiable waste of my life. And frankly, I am inclined to think that it is, for a multitude of reasons, which will serve as the subject matter for my next book(s).

Ten days prior to my writing this sentence, I officially filed for a year's leave of absence from my teaching position at Skyline High School. Where this decision will lead me, I do not know. Time will tell; it always does. In my present state of mind, I have thought the only reason that I might return to teaching chemistry is to try to make some contribution to providing doctors like the ones who saved my life. And I do not mean to suggest that I think only science teachers can help in making such a contribution. Dr. Barnett's high school French teacher, by his own account, was most responsible for his becoming a doctor.

A time or two, I wondered if I had the right to be alive. The way I was looking at things, I had been defective and would not have survived on my own. Medical attention saved me. I had cheated death. Then I got to thinking: Cheating death is the way of life.

If cancer had to happen in our household, I thought it better to have happened to me than to Eva. I do not mean to convey any nobleness in this thought, only an acknowledgement that Eva has known much more physical pain in her life than I have.

Sure enough, too, I had been lucky, very lucky. There is nothing wrong with being lucky, in my opinion. I enjoy telling folks that it is better to be lucky than smart, just so you are smart enough to know when you have been lucky!

I was bound, I suppose, to think about my future sex life. Now that cancer had become part of the equation describing my life, would it derail my interest in sex?

I did think about suicide at various times during my stay at LUH and, in fact, after my return home, too. I do not mean that I ever contemplated committing suicide. But I did give thought to how I would feel about suicide if I found myself in a state of intolerable pain and unacceptable loss of dignity. I prefer to never know a degree of desperation that propels me to ponder suicide. But long before cancer struck me, I argued that the option of suicide is the individual's to ponder, and the individual's alone.

I thought that if I could know that death were coming for me, I would prefer it find me on my terms, in regards to venue. Out of doors and in the morning seem good to me. The season would not matter too much. Locations like my back yard, a beach or a mountain meadow would all serve.

"Huh. All that exercise, and what good did it do me?" was one of my earliest thoughts just after the tumor's discovery. My attitude might have become permeated by bitterness, but Eva rescued my thinking, pronto. She smartly counseled that all those years of rigorous exercise would provide the strength that I would need in the days coming.

Oftentimes, I think back to the time before I knew of my GIST. There I was, blithely living a normal life: working, socializing, planning and so on. All the while, a time bomb was ticking within me. Despite the worsening effects of my anemia, cancer never entered my mind, not even once. One never knows, not really.

Do I now have to feel compelled to spend every waking minute constructively, being somehow productively engaged? Is watching TV a waste of time? How about taking a nap? Should I strive to be outdoors more?

Before this calamity, I used to allow myself to think that I might get to count myself among the lucky ones; the ones fate permits to sidestep serious health troubles, lifelong. Clearly, I have been disqualified from participating in such thoughts.

I do not like to have to think of myself as being among the afflicted. About two months after my surgery, I participated in a cancer-related fundraiser. I did not like doing so. It was very hard. I imagine that I feel like a professional athlete does upon being traded to a team he does not really want to play for, from a contending team to an also-ran. Perhaps I should think, "At least I am still playing."

So far, I have been successful in thinking, "Quit feeling sorry for yourself," when necessary that I do so. Forcing myself to consider those who suffer from some sort of crippling disease or injury helps with my perspective. The woman who declared cancer a dirty word is awaiting a stem cell transplant donor at this writing. Eva and I will dog-sit her basset hound, Otis, for the three months she and her husband must commit to the next round of the fight for her life.

On occasion, I have thought, "Don't talk to me about your medical problems. If you don't have cancer, you're a piker," as someone wants to relate his or her medical story to me. But I would remind myself that we all have our troubles, and we are all made somewhat myopic by them. Obviously, my myopia, if left unchecked, can become putrid with arrogance.

An encounter tending to make one wary is well represented by the idiom, "Once bitten, twice shy." Twice shy, I can handle, if only I can remain bitten just *once!*

Acknowledgements

WRITING THIS BOOK was difficult for me on several levels. I want to thank my wife, Eva, and one of my former students, a young woman named Jenna Borys, for taking the time to proof (several times) my work and for their much appreciated advice and suggestions. Also, a very dear friend and consultant extraordinaire, Dick Mallot, made several valuable points about the book that allowed me to provide the fine tuning and polishing that my work needed. Brian Brown, who is not only my close friend but also my business partner in another venture, was the photographer who shot the photograph for the book's front cover, in addition to offering very valuable help toward the cover's design. Susan Hanes, a dear soul of the highest sort, was a model of patience as I continuously imposed upon her time and expertise while seeking her help in creating the book's cover. Don Cheyne, a wonderful friend, infused me with confidence. Last, but certainly not least, I thank all the good folks who offered me encouragement in my efforts, especially my mother, Mrs. Catherine Irene Gaudio.

About the Author

J AMES J. GAUDIO was born and raised in the Upper Ohio Valley. His hometown is Follansbee, WV, located about forty miles WSW of Pittsburgh, PA. After graduating from high school in 1969, James earned several collegiate degrees, and he has worked in various capacities in the private and public sectors, both as an employee and as a contractor. Upon graduating from the University of Northern Colorado with a BA in Chemistry (emphasis in secondary education) in 1992, James embarked on a new career working as a high school chemistry teacher. During the summer of 1994, he was hired to teach College Preparatory Chemistry at Skyline High School, Longmont, CO. James taught at Skyline until cancer prematurely concluded his school year in April 2007. He and his wife, Eva, continue to reside in Longmont. James is currently pursuing a new career as an author, in conjunction with developing other entrepreneurial interests.